PHARMACOLOGY

A Study Guide
and Self-Evaluation

PHARMACOLOGY

A Study Guide and Self-Evaluation

WALTER H.E. ROSCHLAU, M.D.
Professor Emeritus of Pharmacology
University of Toronto
Toronto, Canada

DEZSÖ KADAR, Ph.D.
Professor of Pharmacology
University of Toronto
Toronto, Canada

B. C. DECKER
AN IMPRINT OF MOSBY–YEAR BOOK, INC.

Mosby Year Book
Dedicated to Publishing Excellence

BC Decker

Editor: Walter Bailey
Developmental Editor: Leslie Fenton
Production Editor: Arofan Gregory
Book Design: Angela Foote
Cover Design: Didona Design Associates

A B. C. Decker imprint of Mosby–Year Book, Inc.

Printed in the United States of America

Mosby–Year Book, Inc.
11830 Westline Industrial Drive, St. Louis, MO 63146

Library of Congress Cataloging-in-Publication Data

Roschlau, Walter H. E.
Pharmacology : a study guide and self-evaluation / Walter H.E. Roschlau, Dezsö Kadar.
p. cm.
Companion v. to: Principles of medical pharmacology. 5th ed. / edited by Harold Kalant, Walter H.E. Roschlau. 1989.
ISBN 1-55664-303-9
1. Pharmacology—Outlines, syllabi, etc. 2. Pharmacology—Examinations—Study guides. 3. Pharmacology—Examinations, questions, etc. I. Kadar, Dezsö. II. Principles of medical pharmacology. III. Title.
[DNLM: 1. Pharmacology. 2. Pharmacology—examination questions. QV 4 R791p]
RM301.14.R67 1992
615'.1—dc20
DNLM/DLC
for Library of Congress 91-24983
CIP

VT/MY/MY 9 8 7 6 5 4 3 2 1

PREFACE

Trends in North American medical education in recent years have shown a drift toward "student-based" learning, generally at the expense of didactic instruction. Combined with ever earlier exposure of undergraduate students to the clinical experience, basic science subjects in medical curricula are in danger of losing their cohesive discipline-oriented identification, and of becoming submerged in as yet unproven educational approaches that are characterized by such fashionable phrases as "student-based learning," "case-based learning," and "problem-solving."

A discernible result of recent curriculum reforms is that many students in the early years of undergraduate medical study find themselves at a disadvantage when required to "learn" a discipline largely on their own (which is the meaning of student-based learning), with the disturbing realization that their basic knowledge may not be sufficiently basic and solid (as a result of case-based learning) to permit true problem solving in the pursuit of complex continuing education.

The "bridging" science of pharmacology has become a tempting target for reform. In some schools it is in imminent danger of being absorbed, as an expedient, by clinical subjects as a "therapeutics" appendix. In several schools it has disappeared from the curriculum entirely. In order to help counteract the erosion, and attendant trivialization, of discipline-oriented pharmacology education, the Department of Pharmacology, University of Toronto, publishes *Principles of Medical Pharmacology* (5th Edition, 1989, edited by H. Kalant and W.H.E. Roschlau). The acceptance of this book as a pharmacology teaching text in North America and abroad has stimulated us to prepare this companion booklet as a study guide and means of self-evaluation for students whose didactic instruction in pharmacology could be superficial or incomplete.

There are several such booklets in circulation that are written with a variety of objectives and question types: problem-solving, judgment, interpretation, factual recall; single or multiple choice from four or five items, matching items, short answers. Most of these publications have a common purpose: to help students prepare for examinations of varying format, rigor, and complexity. So far no other publication provides the rationale for the answers, i.e., helps the learner to learn.

In order to maximize learning and review, this booklet has been laid out in two sections: (1) a *study guide,* loosely coordinated with the sections and chapters of *Principles of Medical Pharmacology,* 5th Edition (1989), the parent text; and (2) a corresponding *collection of uniformly designed questions* for which the given answers are verifiable from the parent text. Thus the study guide represents the organized core knowledge of pharmacology that is needed for entry into clinical clerkship, internship, and for licensing examinations; the questions and answers will indicate to the user the degree of mastery of the subject as well as identify possible deficiencies for correction.

Please note that we have adopted American spelling and usage on the recommendation of the publisher. Where this resulted in significant differences from the Canadian parent text, we have **retained the Canadian equivalent in square brackets [ ].**

Walter H.E. Roschlau, M.D.
Dezsö Kadar, Ph.D.

CONTENTS

SECTION I

STUDY GUIDE

This study guide is based on the chapters of *Principles of Medical Pharmacology,* 5th edition (1989). Because individual approaches to the study of pharmacology differ, and because undergraduate students are frequently overwhelmed by the multitude of seemingly incomprehensible facts, the learning process may derive significant benefit from the assignment of priorities and a clear outline of requirements and objectives. This section, therefore, represents the pharmacology knowledge base (*i.e.,* core knowledge) that is traditionally required of a medical student prior to entry into clinical clerkship, internship, and for licensing examinations. The concurrent use of the parent text will be especially helpful, but many other pharmacology textbooks of recent vintage may prove to be equally good sources of information and instruction.

Each of the chapters is divided under two headings, "Learn" and "Discuss," for interpretation of the subject matter and its priorities.

"Learn" identifies items or topics that require specific and detailed knowledge. Included under this heading are drugs that were chosen on the basis of their relative frequency of use or as important examples of particular classes of drugs. It is normally expected that the factual characteristics (pharmacokinetic profile, pharmacodynamic mechanisms, dose ranges, side effects, *etc.*) of these drugs are known, and that one is able to recall these when pharmacologic problems are discussed and therapeutic decisions are made.

"Discuss" indicates a level of data and knowledge acquisition that can often be accomplished by mobilizing one's biochemical, physiologic, and pathophysiologic background experience in the context of a pharmacologic problem. Learning and understanding these topics in outline may therefore be derivative or integrative. Also included under this heading are less critical facts that may not need to be memorized at once, but that will nevertheless become part of one's total knowledge of pharmacology.

Chapter 1 INTRODUCTION TO GENERAL PHARMACOLOGY

Discuss

Definitions and general principles

Chapter 2 DRUG SOLUBILITY, ABSORPTION, AND MOVEMENT ACROSS BODY MEMBRANES

Learn

Routes of drug administration
Molecular mechanisms of drug absorption
Tissue barriers to drugs

Chapter 3 DRUG DISTRIBUTION

Learn

Volumes of distribution
Sites of drug distribution
Protein binding of drugs
Principles of drug distribution following intravenous injection

Chapter 4 DRUG BIOTRANSFORMATION

Learn

Hepatic phase 1 reactions (with examples)
Hepatic phase 2 reactions (with examples)
Enzyme induction

Discuss

Biologic importance of phase 2 reactions
Nonhepatic sites of drug biotransformation
Variability of biotransformation

Chapter 5 PHARMACOKINETICS

Learn

One-compartment and two-compartment models of drug disposition
Volume of distribution, elimination half-life, and duration of action of drugs
Dosage regimens

Discuss

Principles and measurement of bioavailability
Factors influencing drug bioavailability

Chapter 6 CLEARANCE: THE QUANTITATIVE BASIS OF DOSAGE

Learn

Equations of clearance (Cl), loading dose (L), maintenance dose (D_m), steady state concentration (C_{ss}), and maintenance interval (T_m)
Plateau principle

Discuss

Applications of various dosage regimens; intravenous and oral administration

Chapter 7 DRUG CLEARANCE BY SPECIFIC ORGANS

Learn

Hepatic clearance and first-pass effect
Renal clearance, glomerular filtration, tubular secretion, and tubular reabsorption
Biliary excretion

Chapter 8 DOSE-RESPONSE RELATIONSHIPS

Learn

Properties, uses, and interpretation of log-dose–response curves
Concepts of median effective and median lethal dose
Evaluations of drug safety

Chapter 9 DRUG RECEPTORS

Learn

Nature of biologic drug receptors (with examples)
Concepts of specific and nonspecific receptors

Discuss

Drug-receptor binding: molecular membrane events, cytoplasmic transducers, and cell responses

Chapter 10 SPECIFICITY OF DRUG ACTION

Learn

Molecular basis of stereospecificity (with examples)
Kinetic basis of selectivity
Metabolic basis of selectivity
Interspecies and genetic basis of specificity and selectivity

Discuss

Applications and consequences

Chapter 11 DRUG INTERACTIONS

Learn

Concepts and examples of pharmacokinetic interactions (during the absorption, distribution, biotransformation, and excretion phases of drug disposition)

Discuss

Therapeutic implications and consequences

Chapter 12 HUMAN PHARMACOGENETICS

Learn

Cholinesterase variants
Acetylator phenotypes
Genetic control of P-450 cytochromes
Glucose-6-phosphate dehydrogenase deficiency
Malignant hyperthermia

Discuss

Importance of heredity as a clinically relevant factor in drug efficacy and toxicity

Chapter 13 AUTONOMIC NERVOUS SYSTEM NEUROTRANSMITTERS

Learn

Classification of autonomic innervation
Transmitter substances and their sites of action
Biosynthesis and degradation of acetylcholine and catecholamines
Receptors in the autonomic nervous system

Chapter 14 AUTONOMIC CHOLINERGIC AGONISTS

Learn

Acetylcholine
Acetylcholinesterase
Metoclopramide
Neostigmine
Nicotine

Discuss

Synthetic acetylcholine analogs
Reversible and irreversible cholinesterase inhibitors

Chapter 15 AUTONOMIC CHOLINERGIC ANTAGONISTS

Learn

Atropine
Hexamethonium
Scopolamine

Discuss

Muscarinic receptor antagonists: examples and effects
Nicotinic receptor antagonists (including ganglionic blockers): examples and effects

Chapter 16 ADRENOCEPTOR AGONISTS

Learn

Albuterol [salbutamol]
Dopamine

Epinephrine [adrenaline]
Isoproterenol
Norepinephrine [noradrenaline]

Discuss

Classification and distribution of adrenoceptors
Effects of catecholamines on the various organ systems; metabolic effects
Classification (with examples) of direct and indirect adrenoceptor-stimulant drugs

Chapter 17 ADRENOCEPTOR ANTAGONISTS

Learn

Prazosin
Propranolol

Discuss

Classification (with examples) of α- and β-adrenoceptor blockers
Clinically significant pharmacokinetic characteristics of β blockers

Chapter 18 DRUGS ACTING ON ADRENERGIC NEURONS (ADRENERGIC NEURONAL BLOCKING DRUGS)

Learn

Clonidine
Guanethidine
Methyldopa
Reserpine

Discuss

Clinical significance of adrenergic neuronal blockade

Chapter 19 NEUROMUSCULAR TRANSMISSION AND DRUGS (MUSCLE RELAXANTS)

Learn

Succinylcholine
d-Tubocurarine

Discuss

Cellular events of nerve-muscle transmission
Classification of muscle relaxants according to type of neuromuscular blockade
Clinical importance of neuromuscular blocking drugs and agents acting on excitation-contraction coupling

Chapter 20 DRUGS ACTING ON THE BASAL GANGLIA

Learn

Amantadine
Levodopa

Discuss

Neural connections of the basal ganglia
Basal-ganglion disorders
Approaches to therapy

Chapter 21 ANTISEIZURE DRUGS (ANTICONVULSANTS)

Learn

Diazepam
Phenobarbital
Phenytoin

Discuss

GABA hypothesis of epilepsy
Seizure types
Other drugs in current use

Chapter 22 OPIOID ANALGESICS AND ANTAGONISTS

Learn

Codeine
Meperidine
Morphine
Naloxone

Discuss

Endogenous opioid peptides; distribution in the central nervous system (CNS)

Opioid receptors
Major central and peripheral effects of the opioids
Tolerance and physical dependence

Chapter 23 GENERAL ANESTHETICS

Learn

Enflurane
Halothane
Nitrous oxide
Muscle relaxants (succinylcholine, d-tubocurarine)
Thiopental sodium

Discuss

Types of general anesthesia
Membrane expansion theory
Membrane concentration rule
Classical signs and stages of general anesthesia
Pharmacokinetics of inhalational general anesthetics (importance of solubilities, partition coefficients, and minimum alveolar concentration)

Chapter 24 LOCAL ANESTHETICS

Learn

Lidocaine
Procaine

Discuss

Chemical classes of local anesthetics, structure-activity relationships, relative potencies, and pharmacokinetics
Mechanism of action of local anesthesia

Chapter 25 THE ALCOHOLS

Learn

Ethyl alcohol

Discuss

Metabolic, cellular, behavioral, and endocrine effects of ethyl alcohol
Tolerance, intoxication, and alcoholism

Chapter 26 ANXIOLYTICS, HYPNOTICS, AND SEDATIVES

Learn

Chlordiazepoxide
Diazepam
Phenobarbital

Discuss

Stages of central nervous system depression
Mechanism of benzodiazepine action
Mechanism of barbiturate action
Behavioral effects of benzodiazepines
Adverse effects of barbiturates vs. benzodiazepines

Chapter 27 NEUROLEPTICS (ANTIPSYCHOTICS)

Learn

Chlorpromazine
Haloperidol

Discuss

Classification of neuroleptic drugs
Molecular mechanism of action
Cellular events of neurolepsis
Functional effects of neuroleptics
Adverse effects of neuroleptics and their suggested treatment

Chapter 28 ANTIDEPRESSANTS AND LITHIUM

Learn

Imipramine
Lithium carbonate

Discuss

Types of antidepressants
CNS actions of tricyclic antidepressants (and analogs), monoamine oxidase inhibitors, and lithium ion
Side effects and toxicity of antidepressants (derived from principal actions)

Chapter 29 HALLUCINOGENS AND PSYCHOTOMIMETICS

Learn

Amphetamine
Atropine
Cocaine

Discuss

Structural relationships of lysergic acid, psilocybin, amphetamine, and mescaline families of drugs
LSD syndrome
Amphetamine/cocaine syndromes
Atropine syndrome
Cannabis effects and toxicity

Chapter 30 THE EICOSANOIDS

Learn

Major oxidation pathways of arachidonic acid
Pharmacologic inhibitors of major oxidation steps

Discuss

Role of the eicosanoids in health and disease
Therapeutic uses of $PGF_{2\alpha}$, PGE_1, and PGE_2

Chapter 31 AUTACOIDS

Learn

Pathways of angiotensin, bradykinin, and serotonin formation
Pharmacologic blockers (inhibitors) of angiotensin and bradykinin biosynthesis
Captopril

Discuss

Biologic significance of renin activity, angiotensin II, kinins, and serotonin

Chapter 32 HISTAMINE AND ANTIHISTAMINES

Learn

Cimetidine
Diphenhydramine

Discuss

Types of histamine receptors, effects of their stimulation, and effects of their blockade
Therapeutic uses of H_1-receptor blockers; additional and adverse effects
Therapeutic uses of H_2-receptor blockers; additional and adverse effects

Chapter 33 ANTI-INFLAMMATORY ANALGESICS

Learn

Acetaminophen
Acetylsalicylic acid (aspirin)
Allopurinol
Ibuprofen
Indomethacin
Phenylbutazone

Discuss

Pain, fever, inflammation
Chemical classes of nonsteroidal anti-inflammatory drugs
Major side effects and toxicity (derived from their principal actions)

Chapter 34 DIGITALIS GLYCOSIDES

Learn

Digoxin

Discuss

Physiology of the myocardium; heart failure
Inotropic, electrophysiologic, neural, and extracardiac effects of digitalis glycosides
Digitalis toxicity

Chapter 35 ANTIARRHYTHMIC DRUGS

Learn

Amiodarone
Lidocaine
Phenytoin
Procainamide
Propranolol
Quinidine
Verapamil

Discuss

Mechanisms of arrhythmogenesis
Classification of antiarrhythmic drug action
Additional and adverse effects related to the nature and principal activities of the drugs

Chapter 36 VASODILATORS, ANTIANGINAL DRUGS, AND CALCIUM-CHANNEL BLOCKERS

Learn

Captopril
Diazoxide
Hydralazine
Minoxidil
Nifedipine
Nitroglycerin
Prazosin
Sodium nitroprusside
Verapamil

Discuss

Etiology and pathology of angina pectoris
Pharmacologic effects and side effects of nitrates
Rationale of calcium-channel blockade

Chapter 37 HYPERLIPOPROTEINEMIAS AND ANTIHYPERLIPIDEMIC DRUGS

Learn

Cholestyramine
Clofibrate
Dextrothyroxine
Lovastatin [mevinolin]

Discuss

Lipoprotein transport
Classes of hyperlipoproteinemias
Classes of antihyperlipidemic drugs

Chapter 38 PHARMACOTHERAPY OF HYPERTENSION

Learn

Classification of antihypertensive drugs based on their mechanisms of action (this requires *extensive review* of previous chapters)

Discuss

Specific merits and therapeutic usefulness of diuretics, vasodilators, angiotensin converting enzyme (ACE) inhibitors, centrally acting compounds, and blockers of the autonomic nervous system

Chapter 39 DRUGS AND THE RESPIRATORY SYSTEM

Learn

Albuterol [salbutamol]
Beclomethasone
Codeine
Cromolyn sodium [sodium cromoglycate]
Dextromethorphan
Epinephrine [adrenaline]
Prednisone
Theophylline

Discuss

Bronchial asthma and antiasthmatic drugs
Asthma prophylaxis
Antitussives

Chapter 40 DIURETICS

Learn

Acetazolamide
Furosemide
Hydrochlorothiazide
Spironolactone

Discuss

Renal physiology and major sites of action of diuretic agents
Classification of diuretics (with examples of each class)
Major adverse effects and toxicity of each class
Major therapeutic applications of diuretics

Chapter 41 DRUGS AFFECTING HEMOSTASIS

Learn

Acetylsalicylic acid (aspirin)
Heparin
Warfarin

Discuss

Mechanism of platelet aggregation; pharmacologic inhibition
Blood coagulation; modification by heparin and by warfarin
Therapeutic fibrinolysis

Chapter 42 HEMATINIC DRUGS

Learn

Folic acid
Iron salts
Vitamin B_{12}

Discuss

Nutritional anemias; hematopoiesis
Iron deficiency
Pernicious anemia

Chapter 43 VASOPRESSIN, OXYTOCIN, AND OTHER OXYTOCIC DRUGS

Learn

Desmopressin
Ergotamine

Discuss

Hormonal significance of the hypothalamic-pituitary unit
Physiology of vasopressin and oxytocin
Rationale for therapeutic uses of the hormones and analogs; risks
Ergot alkaloids

Chapter 44 THYROID HORMONES AND ANTIHYPERTHYROID DRUGS

Learn

Levothyroxine
Methimazole
Propylthiouracil

Discuss

Physiology of the thyroid hormones
Hypothyroid and hyperthyroid states
Rationale for therapeutic uses of antihyperthyroid drugs; risks

Chapter 45 GONADOTROPIC AND GONADAL HORMONES

Learn

Basic composition of oral contraceptives

Discuss

Physiology of gonadotropins, estrogens, progestins, and androgens
Pharmacologic control of fertility
Rationale for therapeutic uses of gonadal hormones and analogs; risks

Chapter 46 INSULIN AND ORAL HYPOGLYCEMIC AGENTS

Learn

Chlorpropamide
Insulin
Tolbutamide

Discuss

Physiology of blood sugar control
Insulin preparations
Rationale for therapeutic uses of insulins and oral hypoglycemics; risks

Chapter 47 ADRENOCORTICOTROPIC HORMONE AND ADRENAL STEROIDS

Learn

Beclomethasone
Cortisol (hydrocortisone)
Fludrocortisone
Prednisone

Discuss

Functional relationships in the hypothalamic-pituitary unit and adrenal cortex
Physiology of adrenocortical hormones
Structural (molecular) variations of synthetic analogs
Rationale for therapeutic uses of adrenal steroids; risks

Chapter 48 DRUGS ALTERING BONE METABOLISM

Discuss

Mineral metabolism of bone
Agents with primary and secondary effects on bone metabolism
Rationale for therapeutic uses of these agents; risks

Chapter 49 VITAMINS

Discuss

Fat-soluble and water-soluble vitamins
Signs and symptoms of specific vitamin deficiencies
Rationale for therapeutic uses of vitamins; risks

Chapter 50 PHARMACOTHERAPY OF GASTROINTESTINAL ACID-PEPTIC DISORDERS

Learn

Cimetidine
Omeprazole

Discuss

Physiology of gastric acid secretion
Pharmacologic control of gastric acidity by (a) neutralizing agents and (b) inhibitors of gastric secretion
Agents used to protect the gastric mucosa
Rationale for therapeutic uses of these agents; risks

Chapter 51 LAXATIVES AND ANTIDIARRHEAL DRUGS

Learn

Loperamide

Discuss

Physiology of gastrointestinal motility and intestinal fluid regulation
Classification of laxatives according to their effects on intraluminal fluid accumulation
Rationale for therapeutic uses of laxatives; risks
Rationale for therapeutic uses of opiate analogs in intestinal hypermotility states and diarrhea

Chapter 52 PRINCIPLES OF ANTIMICROBIAL THERAPY*

Discuss

General concepts of antimicrobial chemotherapy; microbial resistance; laboratory monitoring

---

*Note that Chapters 52 to 59 contain references to microbiology, bacteriology, parasitology, and virology that are not strictly pharmacologic but have been included for therapeutic considerations. There is therefore overlap with these other disciplines.

Chapter 53 ANTIMICROBIAL AGENTS THAT ACT UPON BACTERIAL CELL WALL FORMATION

Learn

Ampicillin
Cephalexin
Penicillin G

Discuss

Mechanisms and sites of antibacterial action of the agents in this chapter
Bacterial susceptibility to these agents
Bacterial resistance to these agents
Pharmacokinetics, major adverse reactions, and toxicity of these agents

Chapter 54 ANTIMICROBIAL AND ANTIFUNGAL AGENTS THAT ACT UPON CELL MEMBRANES

Learn

Amphotericin B
Imidazoles
Nystatin

Discuss

Mechanisms and sites of action of agents in this chapter
Microbial and fungal susceptibilities to these agents
Pharmacokinetics, major adverse reactions, and toxicity of these agents

Chapter 55 ANTIMICROBIAL AGENTS THAT AFFECT SYNTHESIS OF CELLULAR PROTEINS

Learn

Chloramphenicol
Erythromycin
Gentamicin
Tetracycline

Discuss

Mechanisms and sites of action in bacterial ribosomes of the agents in this chapter
Bacterial susceptibility to these agents
Bacterial resistance to these agents
Pharmacokinetics, major adverse reactions, and toxicity of these agents

Chapter 56 DRUGS AFFECTING CELLULAR NUCLEIC ACID SYNTHESIS

Learn

Fluoroquinolones
Griseofulvin
Isoniazid
Sulfisoxazole
Trimethoprim

Discuss

Mechanisms and sites of action of the agents in this chapter
Microbial and fungal susceptibilities to these agents
Bacterial resistance to these agents
Pharmacokinetics, major adverse reactions, and toxicity of these agents

Chapter 57 CHEMOTHERAPY OF COMMON PARASITIC INFECTIONS

Learn

Chlorguanide
Metronidazole
Primaquine
Pyrimethamine
Quinidine

Discuss

Drugs used in the treatment of amebiasis, giardiasis, malaria, and toxoplasmosis
Drugs used in the treatment of helminthic infections
Pharmacokinetics, major adverse reactions, and toxicity of the agents in this chapter

Chapter 58 ANTIVIRAL AGENTS

Learn

Acyclovir
Amantadine
Idoxuridine
Vidarabine
Zidovudine

Discuss

General principles of viral replication
Rationale for, and limitations of, therapeutic uses of antiviral agents

Chapter 59 ANTISEPTICS, DISINFECTION, AND STERILIZATION

Discuss

General principles of antisepsis and disinfection
Rationale for, and limitations of, the use of antiseptic agents
Representative examples of antiseptic agents

Chapter 60 ANTINEOPLASTIC DRUGS

Learn

Cyclophosphamide
Methotrexate

Discuss

Principles of cancer chemotherapy
Classification of antineoplastic drugs according to mechanisms of action and sites of action in the cell kinetic cycle
Examples of drugs in each of the major categories
Rationale for, and limitations of, therapeutic uses of antineoplastic drugs
Major adverse reactions and toxicity related to the nature and principal activities of the drugs

Chapter 61 IMMUNOPHARMACOLOGY

Discuss

The drugs named in this chapter and their specialized uses as immunosuppressants and immune modulators

Chapter 62 DRUGS, ALCOHOL, AND THE LIVER

Discuss

Liver functions
Mechanisms of drug-induced liver disease
Mechanisms of alcohol-induced liver pathology

Chapter 63 CARCINOGENESIS AND MUTAGENESIS BY XENOBIOTIC CHEMICALS

Discuss

Chemical carcinogens
Processes of carcinogenesis
Detection of, exposure to, and susceptibility to carcinogens; prevention of carcinogenesis

Chapter 64 CHEMICAL TERATOGENESIS

Discuss

Human risk assessment
Teratologic principles
Pharmacologic principles

Chapter 65 ADVERSE DRUG REACTIONS

Discuss

Classification of adverse drug reactions
Epidemiology of adverse drug reactions
Known examples of adverse drug reactions
Assessment of new drugs

Chapter 66 BEHAVIORAL PHARMACOLOGY

Discuss

Behavioral consequences of drug effects on CNS neurotransmitter activity
Study of drug effects in behavioral models
Study of drug effects on learning and memory

Chapter 67 DRUG ABUSE AND DRUG DEPENDENCE

Discuss

Definitions of addiction, dependence, and abuse
Socially accepted psychoactive drugs
Concepts of behavioral and physical dependence; tolerance
Rationale for, and methods of, treatment

Chapter 68 PERINATAL PHARMACOLOGY

Discuss

Physiology and pharmacokinetic uniqueness of the fetoplacental unit
Perinatal drug disposition; examples

Chapter 69 GERIATRIC CLINICAL PHARMACOLOGY

Discuss

Pharmacokinetic changes in the elderly
Pharmacodynamic changes in the elderly
Principles of dosage requirements and therapeutic implications

Chapter 70 SOURCES OF VARIATION IN DRUG RESPONSE

Discuss

Principles of compliance, bioavailability, and pharmacokinetic and pharmacodynamic variations
Principles of dosage requirements in children and adolescents

Chapter 71 PRINCIPLES OF TOXICOLOGY

Discuss

Toxicants, modifiers of toxicity, and predictive toxicology

Chapter 72 POISONS AND ANTIDOTES

Learn

Chelating agents used in metal poisonings

Discuss

Pharmacologic measures and specific goals of antidotal therapy

SECTION II

QUESTIONS

The questions in this section are numbered by chapter, following the system used in Section I, which is based on the chapters of *Principles of Medical Pharmacology,* 5th edition (1989).

The question format is uniform throughout, employing a popular and versatile multiple-choice model with four items and five options. Question statements are precise and unambiguous, and only one key is required to express the answer to each question as right or wrong.

Key: Answer *A* if 1, 2, and 3 are correct;
B if 1 and 3 are correct;
C if 2 and 4 are correct;
D if 4 only is correct;
E if all are correct.

Of the commonly employed multiple-choice question formats, the one chosen by us appears to be the least objectionable in terms of knowledge assessment, because it permits the testing of factual recall, of problem solving, and of judgmental interpretation. We accept the most frequently expressed criticisms, deficiencies, and limitations of "objective" examinations, which are the apparently rigid formality and the unavoidable simplification of oftentimes complex problems for the sake of quantification of individual responses and statistical analysis of results. Our own studies with large classes have shown, however, that there is no significant difference between multiple-choice, short-answer, essay, and oral assessment when grading individual students on honors/pass/fail and letter scales.

The questions were designed primarily for self-assessment, to instill confidence in one's perceived mastery of the subject, and to identify deficiencies in the traditional knowledge base. The question format requires choosing from unambiguous answers that can be verified objectively in the parent text. By using the answer key as right or wrong, it is possible for users to grade their performance against a standard of individual expectations.

Although the wording of questions varies, each question is expected to be answered in the context of its construction by (1) indicating the correct term(s) or statement(s) from a list of four choices, or by (2) selecting from four choices the correct or most appropriate completion(s) of the lead-in sentence. The answer may then be converted to a letter (A, B, C, D, or E), according to the answer key. The answer will be "right" if the assigned letter is the same as that given for each question in Section III.

GENERAL PRINCIPLES

1–1 Concerning drug nomenclature, which of the following statements are correct?

1. The nonproprietary drug name is also erroneously called the "generic name."
2. The U.S. Adopted Name (USAN) is the official drug name listed in the United States Pharmacopeia (U.S.P.).
3. "Approved" drug names are those recommended for use by national or international scientific bodies.
4. Proprietary names registered by pharmaceutical manufacturers are deliberately chosen to identify the chemical nature of the drugs.

1–2 Drugs used in medicine are conventionally grouped in categories according to their:

1. Source (plant, chemical synthesis, *etc.*).
2. Chemical properties.
3. Potencies.
4. Therapeutic uses.

1–3 Attributes of a "drug" as defined in pharmacology are:

1. An exogenous material applied to, or introduced into, the body.
2. An agent that may be therapeutically useful or toxic.
3. A substance that alters body function(s).
4. A substance required for normal bodily function(s).

1–4 "Pharmacokinetics" deals with (among other things) the:

1. Absorption of drugs from the gastrointestinal tract.
2. Kinetics of drug-receptor binding *in vitro*.
3. Renal excretion of drugs and their metabolites.
4. Biochemical nature of hepatic biotransformation reactions.

1–5 "Pharmacodynamics" refers to the:

1. Quantitative measure of drug effects in the body.
2. Dynamic equilibrium of steady-state drug levels in the blood.
3. Study of the processes affecting fluctuations of drug levels in plasma.
4. Study of the mechanisms of drug action.

1–6 A pharmacopeia is a:

1. Complete list of commercially available drugs, with their uses and dosage forms.
2. List of brand name drugs that have passed independent quality control tests.
3. Periodically updated review of new drugs, with respect to their therapeutic indications and efficacy.
4. Compilation of officially recognized standards of name, purity, potency, and preparation of drugs.

2–1 Continuous constant-rate intravenous infusions of drugs:

1. Guarantee 100% bioavailability.
2. Do not cause a bolus effect.
3. Permit the most uniform maintenance of plasma drug levels.
4. Do not affect the equilibrium between free and protein-bound drug.

2–2 Sublingual administration of drugs:

1. Is the route that provides the highest bioavailability.
2. Does not irritate tissues, as can occur with other routes.
3. Is a suitable means of drug administration in the unconscious patient.
4. Achieves immediate absorption into the systemic circulation, without prior gastrointestinal and hepatic passage.

2–3 Commonly used, effective routes of systemic drug administration include:

1. Oral administration.
2. Intramuscular or subcutaneous injection.
3. Intravenous injection and infusion.
4. Transdermal (percutaneous) administration.

2–4 The first-pass effect in the liver is avoided when drugs are administered by:

1. Inhalation as vapors or aerosols.
2. Intravenous injection.
3. Rectal insertion of suppositories.
4. Deep intramuscular injection.

2–5 Pentobarbital has three more carbon atoms than barbital. Based on this statement alone—and disregarding other factors—it can be predicted that pentobarbital:

1. Is much more slowly absorbed from the gastrointestinal tract than barbital.
2. Needs to be given at 17 times the dose of barbital.
3. Permeates the blood-brain barrier less readily than barbital.
4. Is 27 times more lipid-soluble than barbital.

2–6 As a rule, the majority of drugs will be absorbed across membrane barriers by one or the other of:

1. Passive diffusion through aqueous membrane channels.
2. Active transport *via* membrane carrier molecules.
3. Passive diffusion *via* hydrophobic bonding with membrane lipids.
4. Pinocytosis or phagocytosis *via* the lysosomal system.

2–7 The passive diffusion rate of lipid-soluble drugs depends on:

1. The concentration (or dose) of the drug.
2. The oil/water (membrane/buffer) partition coefficient of the drug.
3. The protonation (= ionization = hydrogen ion concentration) of the drug.
4. The surface area available for absorption.

2–8 The passive diffusion rate of water-soluble drugs across membrane barriers may be determined by:

1. The surface area available for absorption.
2. The concentration gradient.
3. The molecular size of the drug.
4. The availability of an energy source.

2–9 Concerning some aspects of gastrointestinal absorption:

1. The effective pH at the site of intestinal absorption appears to depend on the pH of the intestinal contents.
2. The gastrointestinal mucosa behaves like a lipid barrier in that ionized drugs tend to be poorly absorbed.
3. Drugs with molecular weights greater than 1000 are absorbed by intestinal cells only after breakdown into smaller active substances.
4. Weak bases injected into the bloodstream will appear to be secreted into the stomach and trapped.

2–10 Drug absorption from an intramuscular injection site can be slowed by:

1. Concurrent injection of epinephrine [adrenaline].
2. Application of a tourniquet where feasible.
3. Formulation of the drug with a resin or oil.
4. Exercising the muscle where feasible.

2–11 The blood-brain barrier:

1. Is anatomically characterized by the presence of occluding zonulae between capillary endothelial cells.
2. Is incomplete in the region of the area postrema.
3. Allows the passive diffusion of lipid-soluble drugs.
4. Permits the active transport of amino acids.

2–12 An orally administered weak acid, pK_a 4.0, will:

1. Cause gastric irritation and bleeding.
2. Be predominantly unchanged in the stomach.
3. Have its renal excretion enhanced by acidification of the urine.
4. Exhibit ion trapping inside the gastric mucosal cells.

3–1 A drug's apparent volume of distribution:

1. Is a calculated value.
2. Can be determined by injecting a known dose of the drug intravenously and measuring (by extrapolation) the concentration at time zero.
3. Is the quotient of dose/concentration_0.
4. Allows only rough empiric assumptions of the drug's distribution into identifiable anatomic volumes.

3–2 The sharp fall in plasma levels of a drug within the first few minutes following its intravenous administration is due to:

1. Drug biotransformation.
2. Renal excretion.
3. Biotransformation and excretion.
4. Drug distribution.

3–3 Concerning a drug that is effective both orally (p.o.) and intravenously (i.v.):

1. The drug requires more time to reach the site of action after p.o. than after i.v. administration.
2. The peak plasma concentration is lower after p.o. than after i.v. administration.
3. The drug remains effective for a longer time after p.o. than after i.v. administration.
4. The effect of first pass through the liver would be more important after i.v. than after p.o. administration.

3–4 Concerning possible distributions of drugs in the human body at equilibrium:

1. Mannitol is distributed throughout the extracellular fluid.
2. The distribution of ethanol provides a measure of total body water.
3. Evans blue permits the determination of plasma volume.
4. The volume of distribution of antipyrine equals intracellular water.

3–5 Concerning typical times required for various steps of drug distribution in the human body:

1. It takes about 10 seconds for a molecule of halothane to cross a capillary wall.
2. It takes about 20 seconds for a bolus of fluorescein injected into a cubital (forearm) vein to reach the tongue and the eyes.
3. It takes about 30 seconds for acetylcholine injected into the brachial artery to cause a twitch in the muscles of the hand.
4. It takes about 5 minutes for an intravenously injected bolus of curare to be evenly distributed throughout the plasma.

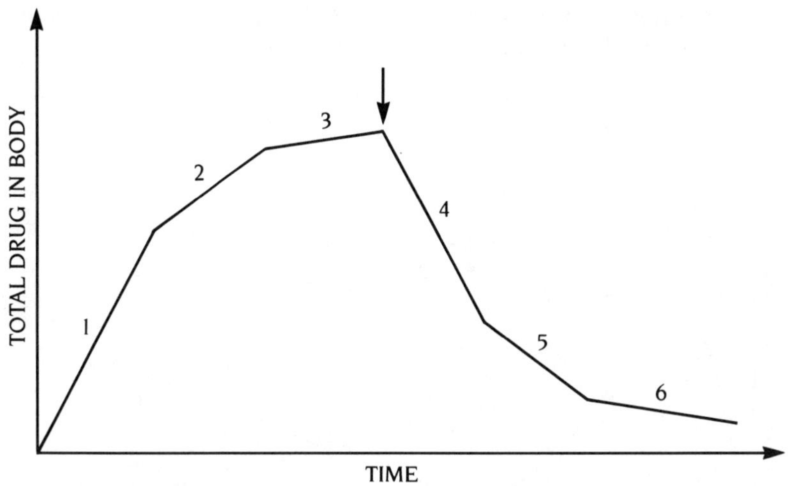

3–6 The graph above illustrates schematically the accumulation of a volatile anesthetic agent in the body during induction of anesthesia and its loss from the body when administration is stopped (*arrow*). It follows that:

1. Total drug in the body is estimated from the cumulative difference between inhaled and exhaled amounts on successive breaths.
2. Segment 1 of the graph corresponds largely to uptake into the heart, brain, liver, and similar organs.
3. Segment 3 largely reflects equilibration into vessel-poor tissues.
4. Segment 4 shows the rapid loss of drug from tissues with poor blood supply.

3–7 The graph below shows schematically the plasma and tissue levels of a drug following a single, rapid intravenous injection.

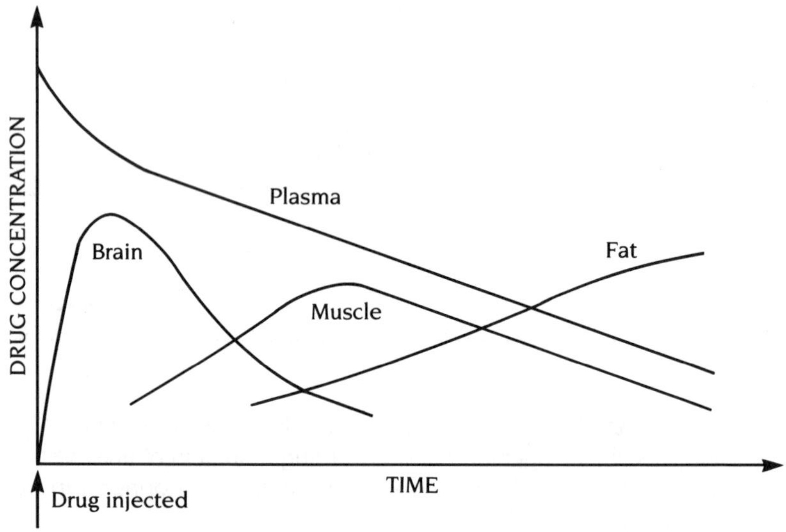

It is concluded that:

1. The high drug levels quickly obtained in brain tissue are most likely due to the relatively large blood flow into that organ.
2. The rapid decline in brain levels of the drug can be explained by redistribution into other body tissues.
3. The drug is likely to have high lipid solubility.
4. The family of curves indicates that the drug is rapidly biotransformed and quickly eliminated from the body.

3–8 Concerning body fat:

1. Adipose tissue is capable of storing large amounts of lipid-soluble drugs.
2. Equilibrium between concentrations of unbound drug in plasma and in fat is quickly achieved.
3. The worldwide use of the insecticide DDT has resulted in its being found in the body fat of nearly all living organisms.
4. Drugs taken up by body fat are excreted *via* the biliary system into the gut.

3–9 Binding of drugs to plasma proteins:

1. Involves mainly binding to albumin.
2. Increases the fraction of drug eliminated by glomerular filtration.
3. Diminishes the pharmacologic activity of drugs.
4. Intensifies (*i.e.*, the bound fraction increases) when the drug concentration in plasma is increased.

3–10 As a result of binding of a drug to plasma proteins:

1. The apparent volume of distribution of total drug may be very low.
2. The fraction of total drug present in unbound form decreases as the drug is eliminated.
3. Displacement by endogenous or exogenous substances may increase the unbound drug concentration.
4. The rate of excretion by tubular secretion is diminished.

4–1 Drug biotransformation:

1. Is the response of an animal organism to a lipophilic chemical.
2. Is responsive to changes in the chemical environment.
3. Can show individual variation on the basis of heredity.
4. Always results in the inactivation of the drug.

4–2 Drug biotransformation is succinctly described as a:

1. Process of oxidation.
2. Process of conjugation.
3. Process of detoxification.
4. Process of polarization.

4–3 Pharmacologic consequences of biotransformation reactions include:

1. Conversion of inactive precursors into active drugs.
2. Conversion of an active substance into another with different activity.
3. Conversion of an active drug into active metabolites.
4. Conversion of an active drug into inactive substances.

4–4 Phase 1 drug biotransformation reactions:

1. Can only occur in mammalian liver tissue.
2. Have as their most active site the hepatic smooth endoplasmic reticulum.
3. Are a biologic necessity for all species of animal organisms.
4. Yield products that are more hydrophilic than the original drugs.

4–5 Phase 1 drug biotransformation reactions:

1. Are catalyzed by the cytochrome P-450 system.
2. Require NADPH, NADH, and molecular oxygen.
3. May be influenced by enzyme induction and inhibition.
4. Require terminal catalysis by cytoplasmic enzymes.

4–6 Induction of the hepatic microsomal cytochrome P-450 system:

1. Is responsible for the more rapid biotransformation of many drugs in smokers as compared to nonsmokers.
2. By ethanol, lacking all substrate specificity for it, has no effect on the rate of oxidation of alcohol.
3. Is relatively specific, depending on which type of inducer is acting and what dose of the inducer is used.
4. By environmental and dietary factors is indicated from controlled laboratory experiments but has not yet been demonstrated in nature.

4–7 Induction of drug-metabolizing enzymes can modify the effects of a drug by causing:

1. An increase in its rate of elimination.
2. A decrease in serum total and free drug concentrations.
3. Reduced pharmacologic effectiveness.
4. Altered pharmacologic activity.

4–8 Phase 2 drug biotransformation reactions:

1. Inactivate the hydroxylation products of almost all drugs that were not inactivated in phase 1.
2. Involve most importantly glucuronic acid and glutathione conjugations.
3. Are subject to certain genetically determined inadequacies in adults.
4. May be temporarily impaired in newborn or prematurely born infants.

4–9 Recognized phase 2 cytoplasmic biotransformation reactions include:

1. Sulfate conjugation of chloramphenicol (catalyzed by sulfotransferase).
2. Hydrolysis of succinylcholine (catalyzed by pseudocholinesterase).
3. Acetylation of sulfonamides (catalyzed by acyl transferase).
4. Oxidative deamination of histamine (catalyzed by diaminooxidase).

4–10 In addition to genetic factors and the influence of age, important variations in drug biotransformation may be caused by:

1. Chronic liver disease, such as cirrhosis.
2. Altered drug distribution as a consequence of renal failure.
3. Thyroid hormone deficiency.
4. High and prolonged fever.

5–1 Patient A may require more frequent administrations of a given drug than patient B, if:

1. Patient A metabolizes the drug faster.
2. Patient A receives higher maintenance doses.
3. Patient A eliminates the drug faster.
4. The plasma protein binding of the drug in patient A is higher.

5–2 The loading dose of a repeatedly injected drug is proportional to the:

1. Required steady-state concentration.
2. Maintenance interval.
3. Half-life of elimination from plasma.
4. Reciprocal of the apparent volume of distribution.

5–3 Concerning a drug with a plasma half-life of 4 hours, given by continuous infusion until a steady-state plasma level has been reached: If the rate of infusion is suddenly reduced by half, then:

1. It will take about a day to reach the new steady-state level.
2. The new steady-state concentration will be half of the previous one.
3. The new rate of drug elimination will be half of the old rate.
4. The drug concentration will decrease linearly with time, and level out at the new steady-state concentration.

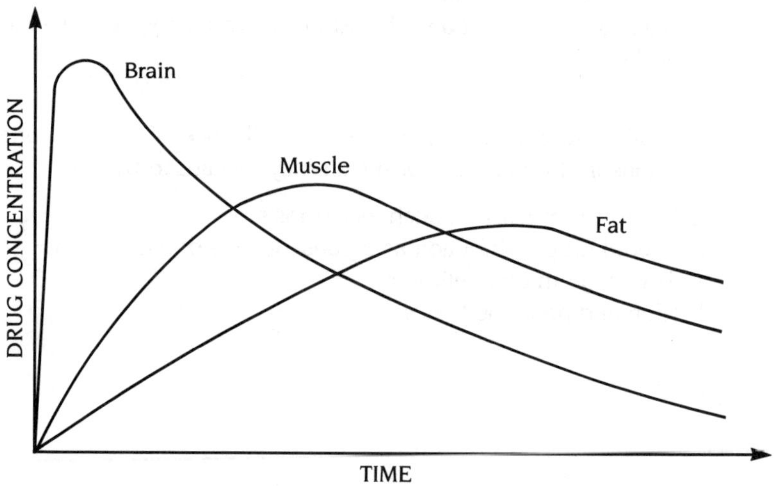

5–4 The graph above shows changing tissue concentrations of a drug in the body. Assuming that the drug does not alter blood flow, the curves could be obtained from which of the following methods of administration?

1. Single oral dose of a slowly absorbed drug.
2. Single intravenous injection.
3. Continuous intravenous infusion.
4. Brief, intensive inhalation of a highly lipid-soluble drug.

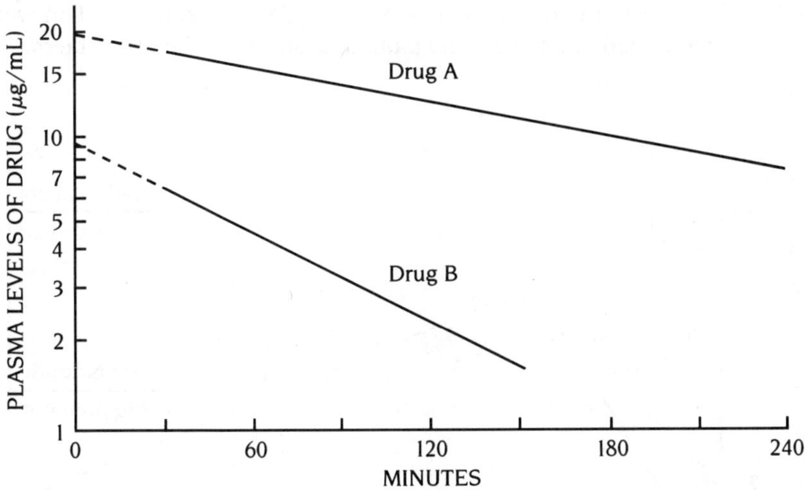

5–5 Concerning two drugs, A and B, given by intravenous injection to men weighing 70 kg each: The dose of each drug was 100 mg. The plasma levels were determined at intervals and were plotted as shown in the graph. From the above data and the plots it can be concluded that:

1. The apparent volume of distribution of drug A is 5 L.
2. Drug A is more likely bound to plasma albumin than drug B.
3. Drug A has a half-life of 180 minutes, drug B one of 60 minutes.
4. The plasma levels of both drugs fall exponentially.

5–6 The plasma concentrations from a single drug administration were determined at intervals and plotted as shown in the graph below.

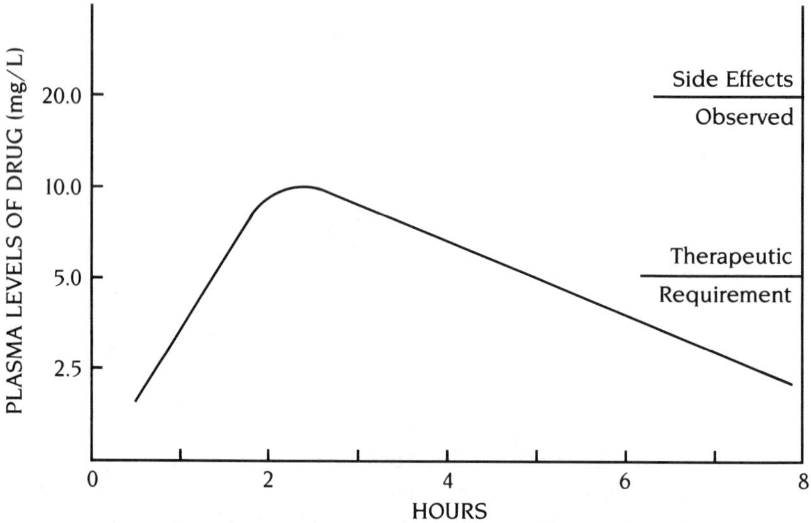

From the above data and the plot it can be concluded that:

1. The drug was administered orally.
2. The apparent volume of distribution of the drug is 5 L.
3. The half-life of the drug is approximately 150 minutes.
4. Readministration of the same dose every 4 hours will provide a steady-state therapeutic plasma level.

5–7 Bioavailability of a drug:

1. Is largely determined by the half-life of the drug.
2. Can be estimated from the area under the concentration-time curve (AUC) after a single drug dose.
3. Is reduced by a high degree of plasma protein binding.
4. Can be markedly affected by the physical properties of the dosage form and preparation.

5–8 Apparent poor bioavailability of drugs may be due to:

1. Slow tablet dissolution time.
2. First-pass biotransformation.
3. Drug interactions.
4. Large volumes of distribution.

6–1 Concerning an exponentially eliminated drug with an apparent biologic half-life of 10 hours: At 10 hours after intravenous administration the plasma concentration is 20 mg/L. From this can be concluded that:

1. At 20 hours after administration, the plasma concentration is 10 mg/L.
2. The apparent initial plasma concentration (C_0) is 30 mg/L.
3. The apparent rate constant of elimination is approximately 0.07/hr.
4. The slope of the line in a plot of $\log_{10}$ (concentration) against time is 10 hours.

6–2 Concerning an exponentially eliminated drug with an apparent biologic half-life of 7 hours and an apparent volume of distribution of 10 L: A dose of 20 mg is injected intravenously into a young man of 60 kg. From this can be concluded that:

1. At 7 hours after administration the drug concentration is 1.0 mg/L.
2. The drug is probably distributed in the extracellular space.
3. The apparent rate constant of elimination is approximately 0.1/hr.
4. Every hour about 7% of the drug still present is removed from the plasma.

6–3 Concerning a drug with an apparent elimination half-life of 10 hours and an apparent volume of distribution of 40 L: Repeated intravenous injections yield an average steady-state plasma concentration of 20 mg/L. From this can be concluded that:

1. A loading dose of 800 mg would establish at once the steady-state concentration regimen.
2. An average concentration of 19 mg/L is reached in 43 hours.
3. An increase in only the maintenance dose interval would reduce the steady-state concentration.
4. An increase in only the maintenance dose would increase the steady-state concentration.

6–4 Concerning a drug with an apparent volume of distribution of 100 L, a clearance of 1 L/min, and a therapeutic plasma concentration of 1 mg/L: When given by intravenous infusion:

1. The loading dose necessary to produce the therapeutic plasma concentration is approximately 100 mg.
2. The maintenance dose necessary to maintain the plasma concentration of 1 mg/L, once it is reached, is 1 mg/min.
3. The steady-state plasma concentration will be closely approached after five half-lives.
4. The therapeutic plasma concentration cannot be reached without first giving a loading dose.

6–5 Concerning an exponentially eliminated drug with a half-life of 2 hours: Following the intravenous injection of a 200-mg dose in a young man of 70 kg, the extrapolated initial plasma concentration (C_0) is 40 mg/L. From this can be concluded that:

1. The apparent volume of distribution is 5 L.
2. A plasma concentration of 5 mg/L is reached in about 6 hours.
3. Strong binding of the drug to plasma proteins is indicated.
4. The drug binds strongly to tissues.

6–6 According to the plateau principle, the time to reach a desired steady-state plasma concentration of any drug, by any route, is approximately five half-lives of that drug. From this can be concluded that:

1. It takes about 4.5 days for phenytoin (t½ = 22 hr) to plateau.
2. It takes about an extra 60 hours to reach a new plateau if the phenytoin dose is doubled.
3. It takes about 7 days for diazepam (t½ = 35 hr) to be eliminated.
4. The levels of steady-state concentrations cannot be changed without also changing the route of administration.

6–7 The graph below represents schematically the time course of drug concentration in the blood of a patient.

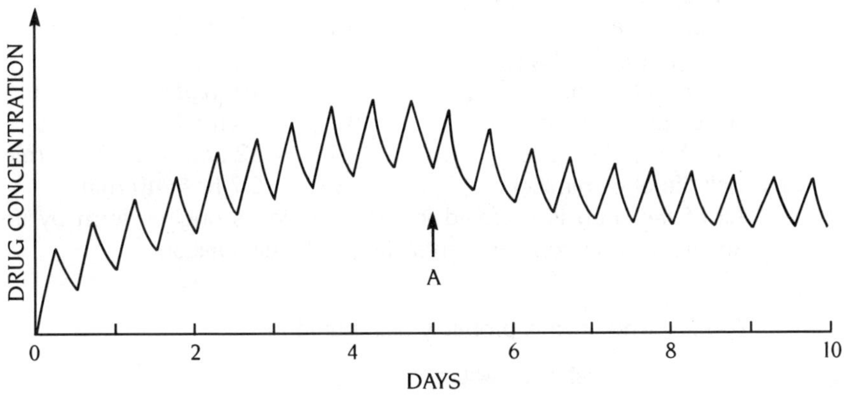

From this can be concluded that:

1. The drug was most probably given in the form of an oral loading dose followed by oral maintenance doses.
2. The half-life of the drug in question was approximately twice the interdose intervals.
3. At point A, a diuretic caused stimulation of drug excretion.
4. Reduction of the maintenance dose by about 40% caused an inflection of the curve at point A.

6–8 Concerning a drug with an apparent volume of distribution of 50 L and an elimination half-life of 3.5 hours, administered to a young man weighing 80 kg:

1. Plasma clearance of the drug is approximately 10 L/hr (≃ 165 mL/min).
2. The drug is probably distributed in total body water.
3. In about 10 hours following a single injection of 200 mg, approximately 25 mg of the drug remains in the body.
4. Drug elimination is by glomerular filtration, but much of the drug undergoes tubular reabsorption.

6–9* A drug is administered by repeated intravenous injections to a young adult man weighing 70 kg. The following clinical and pharmacokinetic data are available:

Therapeutically effective plasma concentration:	C_{ther}	= 5 mg/L
Average steady-state concentration:	$\overline{C}_{ss}$	= 10 mg/L
Toxic concentration:	C_{tox}	= 20 mg/L
Total body clearance:	Cl	= 12 L/hr = 200 mL/min
Half-life of elimination:	$t½$	= 0.7 hr ≃ 40 min

All of the drug is excreted in the urine in its original form by an apparently one-compartmental, first-order elimination.

6–9a The drug is probably distributed in:

1. Total body water.
2. Extracellular fluid.
3. Extracellular fluid, with substantial plasma protein binding.
4. Plasma.

6–9b The drug is probably excreted by:

1. Biliary excretion.
2. Glomerular filtration.
3. Glomerular filtration and tubular secretion.
4. Glomerular filtration and tubular reabsorption.

6–9c The loading dose in the ideal dosage regimen is:

1. 100 mg.
2. 120 mg.
3. 180 mg.
4. 240 mg.

6–9d The maintenance dose in the ideal dosage regimen is:

1. 100 mg.
2. 120 mg.
3. 180 mg.
4. 240 mg.

*Questions 6–9 and 6–10 are pharmacokinetic exercises. Each part has only one correct answer.

6–9e The average rate of drug administration required to reach the desired average steady-state concentration is:

1. 100 mg/hr.
2. 120 mg/hr.
3. 180 mg/hr.
4. 240 mg/hr.

6–9f During elimination following the last administration of the drug, a plasma concentration of 1 mg/L is reached in about:

1. 1.4 hr.
2. 2.2 hr.
3. 3.0 hr.
4. 3.5 hr.

6–10* A drug is administered by repeated intravenous injections to a young adult man weighing 70 kg. The average steady-state plasma concentration to be reached is $\overline{C}_{ss} = 10$ mg/L. The drug is eliminated in the urine in its original form by an apparently one-compartmental, first-order process with a half-life (t½) of 1 hour. The total body clearance is 8 L/hr $\simeq$ 130 mL/min.

6–10a The average rate of drug administration required to reach the desired steady-state concentration is:

1. 80 mg/hr.
2. 100 mg/hr.
3. 120 mg/hr.
4. 800 mg/hr.

6–10b If the drug is injected once every 10 hours, then the doses required to maintain the steady-state concentration are:

1. 80 mg/hr.
2. 100 mg/hr.
3. 120 mg/hr.
4. 800 mg/hr.

6–10c The steady-state concentration would be reached almost immediately by the intravenous injection of a loading dose of about:

1. 80 mg.
2. 100 mg.
3. 120 mg.
4. 800 mg.

6–10d If a 100-mg dose of the drug is injected every hour, then:

1. Immediately before the second injection, 25 mg of drug is in the body.
2. Immediately following the second injection, 125 mg of drug is in the body.
3. The average steady-state concentration is 10 mg/L.
4. At steady state the ratio of maximal to minimal drug concentration is 2:1.

7–1 Total body clearance (Cl) of a drug can be represented as:

1. Cl = (0.693/t½) × total volume of distribution.
2. Cl = dose/$AUC_{0-\infty}$.
3. Cl = total volume of distribution × elimination rate constant (k).
4. Cl = sum of clearances by all organs of elimination.

7–2 The first-pass effect:

1. May cause markedly different pharmacologic effects, depending on whether a drug was given intravenously or by the oral route.
2. For some orally administered drugs may be so pronounced that at low doses no drug will reach the systemic circulation.
3. May give rise to complex and unpredictable drug kinetics.
4. Is a process of drug loss confined to hepatic biotransformation.

7–3 A hepatic drug clearance of 1000 mL/min suggests:

1. High hepatic extraction.
2. Low bioavailability.
3. A strong first-pass effect.
4. A very long half-life.

7–4 Probenecid:

1. Is passively transported from plasma into the tubular urine.
2. Was originally used to prevent the rapid renal excretion of penicillin.
3. Enhances the renal tubular secretion of uric acid in the therapy of gout.
4. Inhibits the active tubular reabsorption of uric acid.

7–5 Important factors in the renal excretion of drugs are:

1. Renal blood flow.
2. Glomerular filtration rate.
3. Renal tubular secretion.
4. Bulk flow of urine.

7–6 Concerning renal excretion of drugs and their metabolites:

1. The concentration of a drug in the glomerular filtrate is the same as the concentration of the free (unbound) drug in the plasma.
2. The tubular reabsorption of drugs involves movement against a concentration gradient, which requires energy.
3. During passive diffusion of drugs from the tubular lumen, the drugs must cross at least two lipidic cell membranes.
4. Only the ionized (charged) molecules of a drug are able to cross lipid membranes during passive diffusion.

7–7 Glomerular filtration of a drug:

1. Is controlled by diffusion.
2. Has a clearance rate of about 220 mL/min.
3. Is slowed by binding to plasma proteins.
4. Is accelerated by enzymes.

7–8 The renal elimination of drugs may be effectively increased by:

1. Administration of a diuretic.
2. Administration of osmotically active substances (*e.g.*, mannitol) excreted through the glomeruli.
3. Alteration of the pH of the urine depending on the pK_a of the drug.
4. Administration of a drug that decreases the plasma protein binding of the drug to be eliminated.

7–9 Concerning pharmacologic implications in biliary elimination of drugs and their metabolites:

1. Drugs eliminated in the bile may undergo enterohepatic circulation.
2. Enterohepatic cycling of a drug can result in its persistence in the body for long periods.
3. Drugs or their metabolites in the bile may be further transformed by intestinal and bacterial enzymes.
4. Biliary clearance is limited to substances having molecular weights of less than 200.

7–10 Concerning drugs that are effectively (highly) extracted by the liver:

1. Their hepatic clearance approaches the total hepatic blood flow.
2. Their hepatic clearance is markedly reduced in the presence of plasma protein binding.
3. Their systemic bioavailability after oral administration may be increased in the presence of severe liver disease.
4. Their hepatic clearance is significantly enhanced by enzyme induction.

8–1 Log-dose–response (LDR) curves:

1. Describe LDR relationships over wide ranges of drug doses.
2. Are typically sigmoidal with a nearly straight middle section.
3. Permit, if parallel, the comparison of relative strengths of different drugs or preparations.
4. Allow the comparison of drugs on the basis of equipotent doses without requiring parallelism.

8–2 The log-dose–response (LDR) curve for an all-or-none (quantal) effect of a drug permits the evaluation of the:

1. Cumulative percentage of subjects responding to a given dose.
2. Dissociation constant (K_{diss}) of the drug-receptor complex.
3. Median toxic dose (TD_{50}).
4. Therapeutic index (TI).

8–3 When all-or-none (quantal) therapeutic and lethal cumulative percentages are plotted against the logarithm of the dose of a drug, parallelism of the resulting sigmoidal curves is not required in order to be able to evaluate the:

1. Median effective dose (ED_{50}).
2. Median lethal dose (LD_{50}).
3. Therapeutic index (TI).
4. Certain safety factor (CSF).

8–4 The relative potency (R) of drug X with respect to drug Y is 2.0, and the maximal responses of the two drugs are identical. From this can be concluded that:

1. The relative potency of drug Y with respect to drug X is 0.5.
2. More drug X than drug Y is needed to obtain the same therapeutic effect.
3. The equipotent molar ratio of drug X with respect to drug Y is 2:1.
4. The therapeutic index of drug X with respect to drug Y is 2.0.

8–5 The bioassay of two drugs produces a graded effect, the log-dose–response (LDR) curves are plotted, and the relative potency (R) of drug A with respect to drug B is 2.0. From this can be concluded that:

1. The LDR curves of the two drugs are parallel.
2. The curve for drug A lies to the left of the curve for drug B.
3. 50 mg of drug A and 100 mg of drug B are equipotent doses.
4. Drug A is safer than drug B.

8–6 The graph below shows the log-dose–response curves of three analgesic drugs.

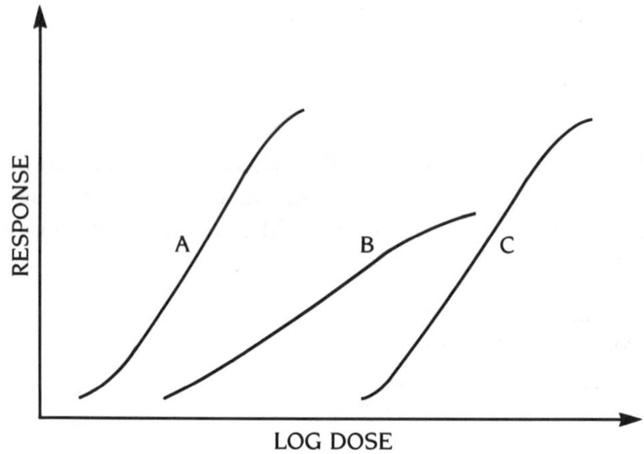

From the plots can be concluded that:

1. The mechanisms of action of drugs A and C are similar.
2. Drug C is less potent than drug A.
3. Drugs A and C are pure agonists, whereas drug B is a partial agonist.
4. The amount at the receptor site of free drug A is less than that of free drug C.

8–7 The dose-response curves for the therapeutic and lethal effects in cats of two drugs, A and B, are shown in the graph below.

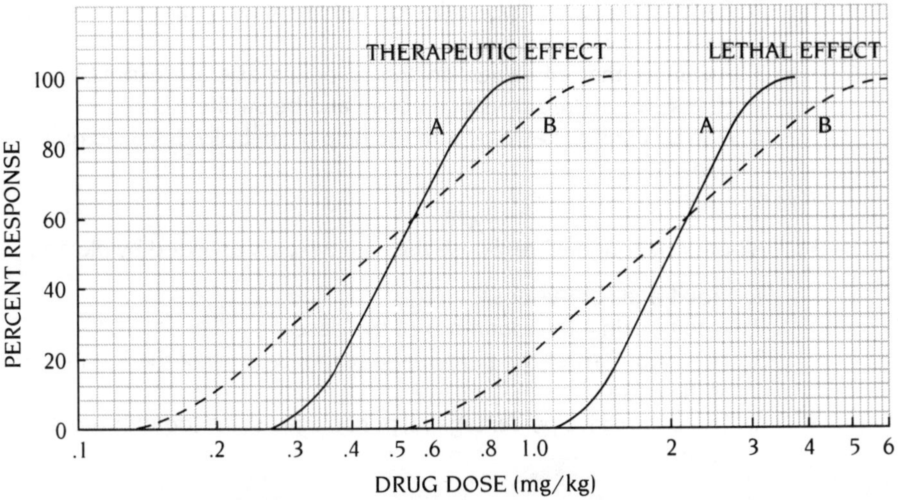

8–7a From this it can be concluded that:

1. The therapeutic index (TI) for both drugs is 4.0
2. The median lethal dose (LD_{50}) for drug A = 2.0 mg/kg and for drug B = 1.75 mg/kg.
3. The certain safety factor (CSF) for drug A is > 1.0 and for drug B < 0.5.
4. The relative potency (R) of drug B with respect to drug A is 1.1.

8–7b Assuming that both drugs are intended for use in human medicine, these observations indicate that:

1. Both drugs elicit a therapeutic effect.
2. Both drugs produce lethal effects at high dosage.
3. Drug A will likely be the safer of the two drugs.
4. The two preparations are pharmacologically similar.

8–8 A probit plot:

1. Is a device to convert a sigmoidal log-dose–response curve into a straight line.
2. Requires the use of log scales for both the x-axis and the y-axis of a dose-response plot.
3. Assumes that all values on the response axis are expressed in terms of standard deviation above and below the ED_{50}.
4. Can be constructed only with the help of specially designed graph paper.

8–9 All-or-none (quantal) response data are typically analyzed by plotting:

1. Probit against the dose.
2. Probit against the logarithm of the dose.
3. The logarithm of the percentage response against the logarithm of the dose.
4. The cumulative percentage response against the logarithm of the dose.

8–10 If the probit response plots for two preparations are straight but not parallel, this implies that:

1. The preparations are chemically unrelated.
2. The therapeutic index (TI) is very low.
3. The ED_{50}s cannot be calculated.
4. The relative response cannot be calculated.

9–1 Which of the following biologic substances may act as specific drug receptors?

1. Membrane enzymes.
2. Membrane sterols.
3. Nucleic acids.
4. Cell proteins.

9–2 Which of the following drug classes require specific receptors for pharmacologic action?

1. Anesthetics.
2. Antibiotics.
3. Osmotic diuretics.
4. Neuroleptics.

9–3 Specific drug receptors can be characterized by:

1. The structure-activity relationships of agonists that cause activation.
2. The antagonists that block the response.
3. The location on presynaptic or postsynaptic membranes.
4. The change in membrane or cell properties accompanying their activation.

9–4 Drug actions that are mediated by specific receptors:

1. Have a threshold dose and a maximum response.
2. Require an energy source for maximum effect.
3. Show positive correlation between potency and stereospecificity.
4. Increase in potency as the drug's membrane/buffer coefficient increases.

9–5 Drugs that do not act through specific receptors usually:

1. Have low chemical structural requirements.
2. Show positive correlation between physicochemical parameters and potency.
3. Must reach high membrane concentrations to be active.
4. Are of low stereospecificity.

9–6 *In vitro* studies of drug-receptor interactions can demonstrate:

1. The affinity of a drug for its receptor.
2. The approximate number of receptor binding sites.
3. The nature of endogenous modulators of the receptors.
4. Whether the drug is an agonist or antagonist.

9–7 Concerning the efficacy of drugs:

1. Efficacy is a measure of a drug's ability to initiate a response when bound to the receptor.
2. Many tissues have "spare" receptors that need not all be activated for a maximum drug effect.
3. Partial agonists cannot produce a maximum response because of low efficacy, even when occupying 100% of the receptors.
4. Efficacy is determined from the height of the maximum response elicited by the drug.

9–8 Many receptors exist in high- and low-affinity states. As a result:

1. A receptor can have different molar affinities for the same agonist, depending on the condition of its existence.
2. The dominance of high- or low-affinity states may be determined by the specific anatomic location of the receptor.
3. Affinity states can be converted from high to low by factors such as sodium ions and guanosine triphosphate (GTP).
4. Susceptible tissues may develop resistance to the therapeutic effects of drugs through changes in the predominant receptor state.

9–9 Concerning effects of drugs on receptors:

1. It appears that drug molecules are capable of changing the conformation of receptors.
2. Drug-induced changes in membrane receptors are directly translated into cell responses.
3. The "occupation theory" implies that a cell responds only for the duration of drug-receptor interaction.
4. The "rate theory" explains the proportionally faster dissociation of antagonist-receptor than agonist-receptor complexes.

9–10 The dissociation constant of a drug for its receptor:

1. Is the concentration of the drug at which 50% of the receptors are occupied.
2. Is usually in the millimolar range.
3. Can be determined by means of radioactive binding assays.
4. Is an accurate measure of a drug's potency.

10–1 Acetylcholine:

1. Shows molecular specificity because the *cis* conformation stimulates only nicotinic receptors and the *trans* conformation only muscarinic receptors.
2. Stimulates nicotinic receptors in both ganglia and neuromuscular junctions, which proves receptor identity in these structures.
3. In linear molecular representation has a distance of 7 Å between cationic and anionic charges.
4. And its analogs (muscarine, nicotine, muscarone, *etc.*) have as a unifying characteristic the free steric rotation of the molecule.

10–2 Stereospecificity is shown by the:

1. l-Form of atropine being the active muscarinic blocker.
2. l-Form of morphine being the active analgesic.
3. l-Form of norepinephrine [noradrenaline] having significant peripheral vascular effects.
4. l-Form of amphetamine being the more effective central stimulant.

10–3 Although used for their predominant molecular differences and specificities, chlorpromazine, procaine, and diphenhydramine share some actions on the basis of common molecular parts. These are:

1. Central stimulant activity.
2. Sedation and dizziness.
3. Antiemetic and neuroleptic effects.
4. Local anesthetic and antihistaminic activity.

10–4 Pharmacokinetic selectivity is shown by:

1. Selective distribution of a drug to a specific target site.
2. Metabolic differences between tissues that result in differential drug activities.
3. Concentration (cumulation) of drugs in excretory organs (*e.g.*, kidneys).
4. Selective distribution of opioid receptors in different parts and tissues of the central nervous system.

10–5 Examples of interspecies differences in specificity or selectivity are:

1. The potential of primaquine to cause hemolysis in individuals with glucose-6-phosphate dehydrogenase (G-6-PD) deficiency.
2. The ability of penicillins and cephalosporins to destroy susceptible bacteria.
3. The damage caused by thalidomide metabolites during the 4th–7th weeks of embryonic development.
4. The relative safety of malathion in birds and mammals.

10–6 Minor structural modifications of sulfanilamide gave rise to specific drug classes, such as:

1. Systemic antimicrobials.
2. Oral antidiabetics.
3. Diuretics-natriuretics.
4. Sedative-hypnotics.

10–7 Examples of selectivity on the basis of human tissue metabolic differences are:

1. The oftentimes greater effect and lower systemic toxicity of anticancer drugs that are injected close to or into the tumor mass.
2. The hydroxylation of cyclophosphamide (antitumor agent) to form free phosphoramide mustard.
3. The ultrashort action of thiopental in brain tissue as compared to other body tissues.
4. The lower concentrations of digitalis glycosides required to inhibit $(Na^+ + K^+)$-ATPase in heart muscle as compared to other tissues.

10–8 Concerning different degrees of specificity or selectivity:

1. Penicillins and cephalosporins are without effects on mammalian tissue enzymes because their action is restricted to the inhibition of a uniquely specific bacterial enzyme in cell wall synthesis.
2. Methotrexate binds strongly to human dihydrofolic acid reductase, which in low doses inhibits rapid proliferation of superficial epithelial tissue, but in high doses has antitumor activity and severe toxicity on all rapidly proliferating tissues.
3. General anesthetics, while acting on many different tissues in the body, exhibit selectivity because of their preferential actions in the excitable membranes of the central nervous system.
4. Cyanide is a poison because of its nonspecific disruption of oxidative metabolism in the mitochondria of all tissues.

11–1 Examples of pharmacokinetic drug interactions are:

1. Inhibition of active renal tubular secretion of penicillin by probenecid.
2. Displacement of warfarin from human serum albumin by phenylbutazone.
3. Induction of hepatic microsomal enzyme activity by phenobarbital.
4. Blockade of nicotinic cholinoceptors by d-tubocurarine.

11–2 Concerning adverse drug reactions on the basis of displacement from serum protein binding sites:

1. Highly protein-bound drugs are more likely to cause these reactions.
2. Increased pharmacologic effects are most marked shortly after administration of a displacing drug.
3. With continued administration of a displacer, the unbound drug concentration returns to normal.
4. This type of drug interaction is the major cause of adverse drug reactions.

11–3 Displacement from serum albumin of one drug by another occurs because:

1. The number of drug binding sites on albumin is limited.
2. Drug binding to albumin is reversible.
3. The binding affinities of highly bound drugs are all about the same.
4. Most drugs bind to the same site(s) on albumin.

11–4 Potential consequences immediately after displacement of a drug from serum proteins are:

1. Increased free drug concentration in serum.
2. Decreased total drug concentration in serum.
3. Increased glomerular filtration of drug.
4. Decreased diffusion of drug into liver cells.

11–5 Potential consequences of induction of hepatic microsomal enzyme activity are:

1. Increased total drug clearance.
2. Decreased serum drug half-life.
3. Decreased serum free and total drug concentrations.
4. Increased rate of production of drug metabolites.

11–6 Concerning the time course to maximum effect of various drug interactions:

1. Induction of microsomal enzyme activity: Days.
2. Inhibition of microsomal enzyme activity: Hours.
3. At the level of receptor interaction: Minutes.
4. Displacement from serum proteins: Seconds.

11–7 Drug interactions may alter elimination rates. Concerning renal excretion:

1. Glomerular filtration of drugs is increased by displacement from serum albumin.
2. Tubular secretion of drugs is decreased by drugs that compete for active transport systems.
3. Tubular reabsorption of weakly basic drugs is decreased by drugs that acidify the urine.
4. Tubular reabsorption of weakly acidic drugs is increased by drugs that alkalinize the urine.

11–8 Drug-drug interactions with potential clinical importance may arise from the combination of:

1. Digoxin and quinidine.
2. Ethanol and barbiturates.
3. Guanethidine and desipramine.
4. Warfarin and salicylates.

11–9 The anticoagulant action of warfarin is reduced by chronic administration of phenobarbital because:

1. The two drugs directly inactivate each other.
2. Phenobarbital competes for warfarin binding sites on serum albumin.
3. Tubular secretion of warfarin is increased by phenobarbital.
4. Phenobarbital induces formation of warfarin-metabolizing enzymes.

11–10 Examples of pharmacokinetic interactions in the gastrointestinal tract are:

1. Improved absorption of some drugs in the presence of increased gastric emptying caused by metoclopramide.
2. Reduced absorption of some drugs in the presence of decreased gastric emptying and intestinal motility caused by opioids.
3. Impaired normal blood clotting from modification of the intestinal bacterial flora caused by broad-spectrum antibiotics.
4. Accelerated and more complete absorption of some drugs in the presence of gastric irritation by ethanol.

12–1 Examples of genetic determination of adverse drug reactions include:

1. Fatal respiratory paralysis caused by barbiturates in persons with acute intermittent porphyria.
2. More frequent peripheral neuropathy caused by isoniazid (INH) among slow acetylators.
3. Excessive β-adrenoceptor blockade caused by metoprolol in poor hydroxylators (SD-defect).
4. Resistance to the anticoagulant effect of warfarin in women of blood groups A, B, or AB.

12–2 Enzymes showing hereditary variations that affect drug responses include:

1. Acetyltransferase.
2. Cholinesterase.
3. Glutathione synthetase.
4. Methemoglobin reductase.

12–3 Drugs that have produced hemolytic anemia in subjects with hereditary deficiency of G-6-PD include:

1. Sulfisoxazole (antibacterial).
2. Acetylsalicylic acid (anti-inflammatory analgesic).
3. Nitrofurantoin (antiseptic).
4. Lidocaine (local anesthetic).

12–4 Concerning hereditary deficiency of G-6-PD:

1. There are hundreds of enzymic variants, many of which are associated with specific biologic events.
2. G-6-PD deficiency in American Blacks gives rise to usually fatal drug reactions.
3. Quinine has caused hemolysis in the Mediterranean, but not in the A^-, variant of the deficiency.
4. In its milder form the deficiency is also known as sickle cell anemia.

12–5 Drugs that are acetylated in the human by the genetically variable N-acetyltransferase include:

1. Hydralazine (antihypertensive).
2. Isoniazid (antitubercular).
3. Phenelzine (monoamine oxidase inhibitor).
4. Procainamide (antiarrhythmic).

12–6 Malignant hyperthermia, a rare inherited muscle disorder, typically is a complication of:

1. Antihypertensive therapy.
2. Frequent blood transfusions.
3. Oral contraceptive use.
4. General anesthesia.

12–7 Atypical cholinesterase, one of the variants of human plasma cholinesterase under genetic control:

1. Occurs in approximately 1 in 200,000 subjects in Caucasian populations.
2. In some families has unusually low affinity for the muscle relaxant succinylcholine, which can enormously prolong the drug's action.
3. Is responsible for most of the treatment failures (*i.e.*, unexpected lack of activity) with ester types of local anesthetics.
4. In some families occurs with threefold higher esterase activity, which renders the muscle relaxant succinylcholine ineffective.

12–8 Genetic susceptibility to hemolytic anemia caused by the antimalarial drug primaquine:

1. Is more common in fast acetylators than in slow acetylators.
2. Results from the genetic deficiency of glutathione reductase in the liver and red blood cells.
3. Can be tested by the addition of primaquine to red blood cells *in vitro*.
4. Is less severe in patients with the A^- variant than with the Mediterranean variant of G-6-PD deficiency.

AUTONOMIC NERVOUS SYSTEM AND NEUROMUSCULAR JUNCTION

13–1 Cholinergic fibers releasing acetylcholine include:

1. Preganglionic fibers to autonomic ganglia.
2. Preganglionic fibers to the adrenal medulla.
3. Postganglionic parasympathetic fibers to effector organs.
4. Postganglionic sympathetic fibers to sweat glands.

13–2 Adrenergic fibers releasing norepinephrine [noradrenaline] include:

1. Preganglionic fibers to the sympathetic trunk.
2. Postganglionic sympathetic fibers to intestinal smooth muscle.
3. Preganglionic fibers to celiac and mesenteric ganglia.
4. Postganglionic sympathetic fibers to effector organs.

13–3 The biosynthesis of acetylcholine:

1. Is governed by the rate of acetylcholine re-uptake.
2. Occurs within cholinergic nerve terminals.
3. Requires extraneuronal acetyl coenzyme A.
4. Is catalyzed by choline acetyltransferase.

13–4 The biosynthesis of catecholamines:

1. Comprises four steps from tyrosine to epinephrine [adrenaline].
2. Occurs in its entirety only in adrenergic nerve terminals.
3. Is rate-limited at the tyrosine hydroxylase step.
4. In chromaffin tissue terminates at the dopamine-β-hydroxylase step.

13–5 Enzymes involved in the inactivation of neurotransmitters include:

1. Acetylcholinesterase.
2. Catechol-O-methyl transferase.
3. Monoamine oxidase.
4. Phenylethanolamine-N-methyl transferase.

13–6 Concerning the criteria required of a true neurotransmitter substance:

1. The precursor substance and the enzyme(s) for neurotransmitter formation must be present in the neuron.
2. The substance must be stored in, and released from, the terminal area when the nerve is stimulated.
3. A mechanism for inactivation of the substance must be present.
4. The effects of endogenous transmitter release must be reproducible by exogenous application of the substance to the effector.

13–7 Norepinephrine [noradrenaline]:

1. Is released upon nerve stimulation from neuronal storage vesicles by exocytosis.
2. At the moment of release constitutes the only substance in the entire discharge from the vesicles.
3. After its release is preferentially taken back into the nerve terminal by active transport mechanisms.
4. Following its re-uptake into adrenergic nerve terminals is methylated to epinephrine [adrenaline] for neuronal storage.

13–8 Sites of metabolic degradation of catecholamines are the:

1. Presynaptic neuronal mitochondria.
2. Presynaptic neuronal cytoplasm.
3. Synaptic clefts.
4. Postsynaptic neuronal cytoplasm.

13–9 Concerning the order of potency of agonists for receptors in the autonomic nervous system:

1. Nicotinic (ganglionic) cholinoceptors: nicotine > carbamylcholine (carbachol) > acetylcholine.
2. Muscarinic cholinoceptors: muscarine > acetylcholine > methacholine > carbamylcholine (carbachol).
3. α Adrenoceptors (α_1 and α_2): epinephrine [adrenaline] > norepinephrine [noradrenaline] > dopamine > isoproterenol.
4. β Adrenoceptors (β_1 and β_2): isoproterenol > epinephrine [adrenaline] > norepinephrine [noradrenaline] > dopamine.

13–10 Concerning modulation of autonomic nervous system activity:

1. Drug-induced elevation of mean arterial pressure may cause bradycardia through baroreceptor stimulation and cholinergic predominance.
2. Presynaptic α_2-adrenoceptor stimulation by an agonist may cause reduction of norepinephrine [noradrenaline] release through negative feedback control.
3. Prolonged excessive stimulation of adrenoceptors may cause desensitization due to down-regulation (*i.e.,* decreased receptor numbers).
4. Endogenous prostaglandins, enkephalins, and angiotensin II may enhance the release of norepinephrine [noradrenaline] through inhibition of presynaptic adrenoceptors.

14–1 The muscarinic actions of acetylcholine include:

1. Stimulation of exocrine glands, including (in part) gastric and intestinal secretions.
2. Contraction of smooth muscles in bronchi, gastrointestinal tract, and gall and urinary bladders.
3. Contraction of circular muscles of the iris and the muscles of accommodation.
4. Relaxation of sphincters in gastrointestinal, biliary, and urinary tracts.

14–2 Direct nicotinic actions of acetylcholine include:

1. Contraction of skeletal muscles.
2. Stimulation of autonomic ganglia.
3. Stimulation of catecholamine release from the adrenal medulla.
4. Slowing of the heart rate (bradycardia).

14–3 Synthetic analogs of acetylcholine:

1. Indirectly stimulate the release of acetylcholine from cholinergic neurons.
2. Have greater resistance than acetylcholine to cholinesterase hydrolysis (*e.g.*, carbamylcholine).
3. Are designed for use in conditions where the "natural" cholinergic drugs are contraindicated (*e.g.*, intestinal or urinary obstruction).
4. Can have more selectively muscarinic activity relative to nicotinic actions (*e.g.*, methacholine).

14–4 Acetylcholinesterase inhibitors:

1. Inhibit both acetylcholinesterase and plasma cholinesterase, although to varying extents.
2. Consist of two chemical classes of compounds: carbamates and organophosphates.
3. Have pharmacologic effects only in organ structures in which acetylcholine is a neurotransmitter.
4. Have shown significant variability in response in the presence of "atypical acetylcholinesterase."

14–5 Concerning reversible cholinesterase inhibitors:

1. Physostigmine, a tertiary nitrogen compound, can cross the blood-brain barrier.
2. Neostigmine, a quaternary nitrogen compound, has some direct action on nicotinic receptors in skeletal muscle.
3. Edrophonium, a short-acting compound, is used in the differential diagnosis of myasthenia gravis.
4. Ambenonium, an ultra-short-acting quaternary ammonium compound, has no central nervous system–related side effects.

14–6 Irreversible cholinesterase inhibitors:

1. Are strong poisons without beneficial properties for use in medicine.
2. Phosphorylate the esteratic site of acetylcholine.
3. Are not strictly irreversible because the covalent interaction of aged phosphorylation can be reversed and the enzyme reactivated with pralidoxime (2-PAM).
4. Are the basis of many insecticides because of the much more rapid activation in insects than in mammals of thiophosphates to phosphates.

14–7 Metoclopramide:

1. Is a dopamine antagonist with indirect cholinergic activity.
2. In the alimentary tract produces all effects of direct cholinergic stimulation.
3. Has strong central antiemetic properties.
4. Facilitates rapid healing of gastric ulcers.

14–8 Concerning the effects of nicotine on organ systems:

1. Small doses act on chemoreceptors in aortic and carotid bodies, resulting in depression of respiration.
2. Higher doses stimulate autonomic ganglia, which produces the characteristic tremor and nausea.
3. The acute intake of toxic amounts paralyzes the medulla oblongata, with death due to respiratory failure.
4. Chronic intoxication may lead to serious circulatory defects in susceptible vascular beds.

15–1 Atropine:

1. Is a naturally occurring plant alkaloid, dl-hyoscyamine, extracted from species of the potato family.
2. Is a specific muscarinic cholinoceptor blocker.
3. Applied locally in the form of eyedrops causes mydriasis and cycloplegia.
4. In high doses has complicated effects on the brain, which are generally stimulatory and disorienting.

15–2 Scopolamine:

1. Is a synthetic cholinergic muscarinic antagonist.
2. Is qualitatively identical to atropine in its peripheral and central actions.
3. Is the preferred anticholinergic agent to treat gastrointestinal disorders.
4. Is used prophylactically to prevent motion sickness.

15–3 Synthetic muscarinic antagonists were developed to maximize specific actions of atropine, such as:

1. Suppression of gastric secretions in gastric ulcer therapy (*e.g.*, pirenzepine).
2. Relaxation of uterine muscle in premature labor (*e.g.*, dicyclomine).
3. Symptomatic (adjunctive) treatment of Parkinson's disease (*e.g.*, benztropine).
4. Ganglionic blockade to treat hypertensive crisis (*e.g.*, trimethaphan).

15–4 The effects of ganglionic blockade with hexamethonium on various organs include:

1. Dilatation of the pupils.
2. Disturbed intestinal motility and constipation.
3. Dry and flushed skin.
4. Mental confusion and hallucinations.

15–5 Nicotinic receptors in autonomic ganglia:

1. Are structurally identical to nicotinic receptors at neuromuscular junctions.
2. Will be blocked by bisquaternary ammonium compounds having five- or six-carbon bridges.
3. Respond differently to various blocking agents because of differences between sympathetic and parasympathetic ganglia.
4. When blocked will alter organ functions, depending on that system's dominant tone (sympathetic:parasympathetic).

16–1 Drugs classified as sympathomimetics include those that:

1. Directly stimulate α and/or β adrenoceptors, and/or dopamine receptors.
2. Increase the release of neurotransmitter from sympathetic nerve terminals.
3. Block the re-uptake of neurotransmitter by adrenergic neurons.
4. Accelerate the intraneuronal synthesis of neurotransmitter.

16–2 Which of the catecholamines are agonists (although with differing affinities) at all known adrenoceptor types (α_1, α_2, β_1, β_2)?

1. Dopamine.
2. Norepinephrine [noradrenaline].
3. Isoproterenol.
4. Epinephrine [adrenaline].

16–3 Concerning the significance of -OH groups in the catecholamine structure:

1. The hydroxyl groups in the C-3 and C-4 positions of the benzene ring confer characteristic α- and β-adrenergic activity.
2. A hydroxyl group on the α carbon in the side chain allows very rapid oxidation by monoamine oxidase.
3. A hydroxyl group on the β carbon in the side chain enhances direct adrenoceptor-stimulant action.
4. Addition of a third -OH group in the C-5 position of the benzene ring converts the molecule from an agonist into an antagonist.

16–4 Concerning the molecular effects of adrenoceptor stimulation:

1. Stimulation of α_1 adrenoceptors causes membranal synthesis of intracellular messengers inositol triphosphate and diacylglycerol.
2. Stimulation of (postsynaptic) α_2 adrenoceptors inhibits adenylate cyclase, with consequent lowering of intracellular cyclic AMP.
3. Stimulation of β adrenoceptors raises the concentration of intracellular cyclic AMP for combination with a protein kinase.
4. Stimulation of postsynaptic adrenoceptors (and the subsequent molecular events) by sympathomimetic drugs requires an intact sympathetic innervation.

16–5 The stimulation by catecholamines of β_1 adrenoceptors in the heart produces:

1. Positive inotropic effects.
2. Positive chronotropic effects.
3. Increased consumption of oxygen.
4. Occasional arrhythmias.

16–6 Concerning vascular effects of catecholamines:

1. Norepinephrine [noradrenaline] constricts all blood vessels, which increases total peripheral vascular resistance.
2. Low doses of epinephrine [adrenaline] cause vasoconstriction in skin, mucous membranes, and kidneys, but vasodilatation in skeletal muscles.
3. Isoproterenol lowers peripheral vascular resistance, with consequent fall in diastolic blood pressure.
4. Vasoconstrictor effects of dopamine are dose-dependent: low doses stimulate α adrenoceptors, while high doses stimulate dopamine receptors.

16–7 Concerning catecholamine-induced metabolic and endocrine effects:

1. Reduction of lipase activity impedes the breakdown of triglycerides to glycerol and fatty acids.
2. Increased glycogen storage in the liver may cause hypoglycemia.
3. Gluconeogenesis from lactate and amino acids is blocked.
4. Insulin release from pancreatic islet cells is inhibited by α-adrenoceptor stimulants.

16–8 Selective α_1-adrenoceptor agonists in clinical use:

1. Have actions that are very similar to epinephrine [adrenaline].
2. Are used primarily for their vasoconstrictor effects.
3. All have very short durations of action.
4. May cause vagal bradycardia mediated by baroreceptor stimulation.

16–9 Selective β_2-adrenoceptor agonists in clinical use:

1. Have weak myocardial stimulating properties.
2. Are used primarily for their bronchodilator action.
3. Relax the pregnant uterus.
4. Decrease peripheral vascular resistance.

16–10 Ephedrine:

1. Enhances the release of norepinephrine [noradrenaline] from sympathetic nerve endings.
2. Shows greater sympathomimetic activity when used as the dextrorotatory isomer.
3. Has direct stimulating effects on α_1, β_1, and β_2 adrenoceptors.
4. Has vasopressor activity that is 7–10 times greater than that of epinephrine [adrenaline].

16–11 Which of the following correctly describe the listed drugs' mechanisms of action and effects on the adrenergic system?

1. Cocaine	Blocks neurotransmitter re-uptake.	Extracellular accumulation of neurotransmitter and potentiation of response.
2. Amphetamine	Displaces neurotransmitter from nerve terminals.	Indirect sympathomimetic effect.
3. Phenylephrine	Mimics neurotransmitter at postsynaptic receptors.	Direct sympathomimetic effect.
4. α-Methyldopa	Transforms into (false) neurotransmitter.	Blockade of normal transmitter release.

17–1 Concerning α-adrenoceptor antagonists:

1. The receptor blockade by phenoxybenzamine is irreversible and persists for several days after a single dose.
2. The α_2-adrenoceptor blockade by phentolamine causes severe bradycardia in addition to peripheral vasodilatation.
3. Prazosin, because of its selective α_1-adrenoceptor blockade, is used clinically to treat essential hypertension.
4. Tolazoline, a reversible α-adrenoceptor blocker, is used mainly as an oral antidiabetic agent.

17–2 So-called cardioselective β blockers include:

1. Atenolol.
2. Esmolol.
3. Metoprolol.
4. Labetalol.

17–3 Nonselective β blockers (prototype propranolol):

1. Are competitive antagonists of endogenous catecholamines and exogenous sympathomimetic drugs that act on β adrenoceptors.
2. Cause a profound decrease in peripheral vascular resistance, which is the rationale for their use in the treatment of hypertension.
3. Increase airway resistance and may cause bronchospasm in asthmatic individuals.
4. Are contraindicated in diabetics because they inactivate injected insulin, causing uncontrollable hyperglycemia.

17–4 Pharmacokinetic characteristics of propranolol include:

1. Rapid and complete absorption from the gastrointestinal tract.
2. Extensive first-pass transformation resulting in poor bioavailability.
3. Production of an active metabolite.
4. Binding to plasma proteins in excess of 90%.

17–5 Indications for the therapeutic use of β blockers include:

1. Raynaud's disease.
2. Essential hypertension.
3. Preoperative management of pheochromocytoma.
4. Thyrotoxicosis.

17–6 The specific cardiac effects of propranolol (and other β blockers) include:

1. Bradycardia.
2. Reduced cardiac output.
3. Decreased automaticity of pacemaker cells.
4. Increased myocardial oxygen consumption.

18–1 Reserpine:

1. Is a natural plant alkaloid.
2. Depletes central and peripheral stores of catecholamines and serotonin.
3. Has antihypertensive actions primarily because of norepinephrine [noradrenaline] depletion.
4. Can cause receptor supersensitivity to catecholamines and direct-acting sympathomimetics.

18–2 Adverse reactions to reserpine include:

1. Bradycardia, nasal congestion, and postural hypotension.
2. Depression of mood and possible parkinsonism.
3. Increased secretion of prolactin and occasional galactorrhea.
4. Reduced gastric acid secretion and gastrointestinal motility.

18–3 Guanethidine:

1. Produces its pharmacologic effects primarily through impairment of neurotransmitter release.
2. Action is unaffected by the presence of drugs that block the uptake of norepinephrine [noradrenaline].
3. Has a prolonged action when used in the treatment of hypertension, its principal therapeutic use.
4. Readily crosses the blood-brain barrier, with adverse effects on brain catecholamines.

18–4 Concerning α-methyldopa:

1. The drug is converted to α-methylnorepinephrine [α-Me-noradrenaline] (a "false" transmitter) in central and peripheral neurons.
2. The "false" transmitter is released together with norepinephrine [noradrenaline] from terminal varicosities.
3. α-Methylnorepinephrine stimulates (postsynaptic) α_2 adrenoceptors in the central nervous system, inhibiting peripheral neurotransmitter release.
4. In peripheral nerves the released α-methylnorepinephrine acts as a blocker of α_1 adrenoceptors.

18–5 The enzymes involved in the conversion of α-methyldopa to α-methylnorepinephrine [α-Me-noradrenaline] are:

1. Tyrosine hydroxylase.
2. Dopa decarboxylase.
3. Monoamine oxidase.
4. Dopamine-β-hydroxylase.

18–6 Clonidine:

1. Is classified as a (presynaptic) α_2-adrenoceptor stimulant.
2. Causes a reduction of norepinephrine [noradrenaline]release from sympathetic neurons.
3. Lowers blood pressure by a combination of bradycardia and reduced cardiac output.
4. May cause "rebound" hypertension when suddenly withdrawn.

19–1 The release of acetylcholine in neuromuscular junctions:

1. Occurs in response to a somatic nerve action potential.
2. Is part of a cycle of events that requires only seconds to complete.
3. Requires fusion of cytoplasmic acetylcholine vesicles with the presynaptic membrane.
4. Is followed by cytoplasmic synthesis of new acetylcholine within cisterns formed from empty vesicles.

19–2 Endplate potentials in neuromuscular junctions:

1. Are the result of interaction of released acetylcholine molecules with nicotinic receptors on the muscle cell membrane (sarcolemma).
2. Are graded events that depend on the number of acetylcholine molecules available for receptor interaction.
3. Are accompanied by ion fluxes, *via* postsynaptic ionophores, of Na^+, K^+, and Cl^-.
4. Cause depolarization of membranes of the sarcoplasmic reticulum, the release of Ca^{2+}, and muscle contraction.

19–3 Acetylcholine release from vesicles in prejunctional nerve terminals:

1. May be prevented to a degree by local and general anesthetics that block the nerve impulse.
2. Is greatly stimulated by ethanol concentrations in body water of > 40 mM, as, for example, in severe alcohol intoxication.
3. Is blocked by botulinum toxin, which will cause death in very low concentrations.
4. Is greatly reduced by black widow spider venom, causing temporary paralysis and flaccidity of skeletal muscles.

19–4 d-Tubocurarine:

1. Is a competitive nondepolarizing nicotinic receptor blocker at neuromuscular junctions.
2. Competes with acetylcholine for receptor sites because of its bisquaternary ammonium structure and rigid molecular configuration.
3. Has zero efficacy and can be removed from the receptors by increasing the concentrations of acetylcholine.
4. In high doses will cause cardiac arrest from paralysis of the myocardium.

19–5 Clinically encountered untoward effects of d-tubocurarine are:

1. Abnormally delayed elimination by slow acetylators.
2. Transient hypotension caused by the release of histamine.
3. Convulsive seizures caused by CNS irritation.
4. Transient apnea caused by paralysis of respiratory muscles.

19–6 Succinylcholine:

1. Has an acetylcholine-like structure and acts like an excess of transmitter in the neuromuscular synaptic cleft.
2. Causes depolarization and desensitization of nicotinic receptors, which are preceded by muscle fasciculation.
3. Is hydrolyzed by plasma cholinesterase, of which there are genetic variants.
4. Does not cause apnea because of its rapid onset and short duration of action.

19–7 Clinical uses of succinylcholine include:

1. The specific treatment of malignant hyperthermia.
2. The specific treatment of myasthenia gravis.
3. Reversal of the effects of d-tubocurarine overdose.
4. Muscle relaxation (*e.g.*, general anesthesia; electroconvulsive therapy).

CENTRAL NERVOUS SYSTEM

20–1 The basal ganglia include the:

1. Caudate-putamen (striatum).
2. Substantia nigra.
3. Globus pallidus.
4. Thalamus.

20–2 Functionally important transmitter substances in neurons of the caudate-putamen–substantia nigra pathways include:

1. Acetylcholine.
2. Dopamine.
3. Gamma-aminobutyric acid (GABA).
4. Glutamate.

20–3 The crucial anatomic change found in parkinsonian brains is progressive cell loss in the:

1. Caudate-putamen.
2. Globus pallidus.
3. Subthalamus.
4. Substantia nigra.

20–4 In terms of biochemical changes in the caudate-putamen, the parkinsonian syndrome arises from a relative:

1. Decrease in GABA levels.
2. Reduction of dopamine content.
3. Loss of acetylcholine neurons.
4. Acetylcholine predominance.

20–5 Concerning pharmacologic approaches to the treatment of parkinsonism:

1. Amantadine increases dopamine release from nigral neurons.
2. Cholinergic muscarinic antagonists tend to restore a functional dopamine-acetylcholine balance.
3. Dopamine mimetics may stimulate dopamine receptors directly.
4. Inhibition of monoamine oxidase B raises dopamine levels by preventing its breakdown.

20–6 Levodopa:

1. Is a precursor of dopamine.
2. Easily crosses the blood-brain barrier.
3. Causes increased dopamine output in parkinsonian brains.
4. Is only effective in the presence of dopamine-producing neurons.

20–7 Carbidopa:

1. Is a peripheral decarboxylase inhibitor.
2. Has effects on the brain similar to those of levodopa.
3. Reduces the systemic side effects of levodopa when given together.
4. Slows down the catabolism of dopamine.

20–8 Concerning Huntington's chorea:

1. The predominant symptoms are hyperkinesia and progressive mental deterioration.
2. The biochemical basis is a degenerative reduction of GABA and acetylcholine in the caudate-putamen.
3. Choretic movements respond to dopamine receptor blockers (*e.g.*, neuroleptics) and restoration of the dopamine-acetylcholine balance.
4. Raising GABA activity with GABA agonists (*e.g.*, progabide) effectively counteracts the dementia of the disease.

21–1 Different epileptic seizure types respond differently to antiseizure drugs. For example:

1. Ethosuximide is currently the drug of choice for absence (petit mal) seizures.
2. Unless accompanied by annoying side effects, tonic-clonic (grand mal) attacks are treated with phenytoin.
3. Status epilepticus is quickly terminated with intravenously administered diazepam.
4. Carbamazepine is the preferred drug against complex partial (psychomotor, temporal lobe) seizures.

21–2 Well-known disadvantages of phenytoin include:

1. Frequent hirsutism and gingival hyperplasia.
2. Marked sedation at therapeutic dose levels.
3. Sudden changes of metabolic processes within the therapeutic range of plasma concentrations.
4. Personality changes in up to 50% of treated patients.

21–3 Gastrointestinal disturbances as a drug side effect can be expected with the use of:

1. Ethosuximide.
2. Valproate.
3. Carbamazepine.
4. Phenobarbital.

21–4 Unacceptably high (toxic) phenobarbital serum levels may occur as a consequence of drug-drug interaction with:

1. Diazepam.
2. Primidone.
3. Phenytoin.
4. Valproate.

21–5 Gamma-aminobutyric acid (GABA):

1. Is an inhibitory neurotransmitter in many parts of the central nervous system.
2. Is synthesized from L-glutamic acid by L-glutamic acid decarboxylase (GAD).
3. Is broken down by α-ketoglutarate-GABA transaminase (GABA-T).
4. Acts on macromolecular $GABA_A$ receptors containing chloride channels.

21–6 Concerning GABA receptors:

1. Antagonists for $GABA_A$ receptors have convulsant properties.
2. Benzodiazepines, by interfering with $GABA_A$ receptors, block Cl^- movements through ionophores.
3. The effects of specific $GABA_A$-receptor activation are of an antispastic nature.
4. GABA receptors in the spinal cord and lower brain stem act as specific glycine recognition sites.

22–1 Opioids of the phenanthrene class include:

1. Morphine.
2. Thebaine.
3. Heroin.
4. Papaverine.

22–2 Opioid-receptor binding is:

1. Structurally specific.
2. Stereospecific.
3. Competitive.
4. Reversible.

22–3 Opioid receptors exist in various types as exclusive binding sites for prototypical ligands, such as:

1. μ Receptors for β-endorphin.
2. κ Receptors for naloxone.
3. δ Receptors for met-enkephalin.
4. σ Receptors for morphine.

22–4 Concerning the analgesia produced by morphine:

1. Pain tolerance is increased more than pain threshold.
2. Morphine is more effective against sharp, intermittent pain than against dull, constant pain.
3. The analgesic effect is enhanced by mental clouding and detachment.
4. The analgesia is not prevented or reversed by narcotic antagonists.

22–5 Fundamental central effects of morphine include:

1. Analgesia.
2. Changes in mood.
3. Respiratory depression.
4. Sedation.

22–6 Peripheral and endocrine effects of opioids include:

1. Antidiuresis.
2. Histamine release.
3. Smooth muscle contraction.
4. Nausea and vomiting.

22–7 Morphine and meperidine are similar in:

1. Analgesic potency.
2. Addiction liability.
3. Causing miosis.
4. Depressing respiration.

22–8 Morphine and methadone are similar in:

1. Analgesic potency.
2. Intensity of euphoria.
3. Causing miosis.
4. Duration of action.

22–9 Addicts appear to prefer heroin over other opiates because:

1. Heroin is much less toxic than morphine.
2. Heroin does not cause miosis.
3. Heroin does not depress respiration.
4. Heroin has a rapid onset of action.

22–10 Pure morphine antagonists include:

1. Buprenorphine.
2. Naltrexone.
3. Pentazocine.
4. Naloxone.

23–1 The "classical" stages of general anesthesia are characterized as follows:

1. Stage I = analgesia as a consequence of blockade of neurons in lamina 4 of the dorsal horn in the spinal cord.
2. Stage II = delirium and excitement as a consequence of blockade of small inhibitory cells of the Golgi type II.
3. Stage III = surgical anesthesia as a consequence of progressive depression of the brain stem reticular systems.
4. Stage IV = imminent death as a consequence of paralysis of the respiratory and vasomotor centers in the medulla oblongata.

23–2 The mode of action of general anesthetics is believed to involve:

1. An expansion of excitable cell membranes.
2. A decrease in sodium channel conductance.
3. An increase in the firing threshold of the nerve cell.
4. An increase in the rate of rise of the action potential.

23–3 Clinically acceptable general anesthesia (so-called balanced anesthesia) should be capable of providing:

1. Hypnosis.
2. Analgesia.
3. Amnesia.
4. Hemostasis.

23–4 Atropine is routinely employed during general anesthesia in order to:

1. Sedate the patient prior to induction of anesthesia.
2. Reduce salivary and respiratory tract secretions.
3. Induce muscular relaxation through cholinergic receptor blockade.
4. Block vagal reflexes.

23–5 The speed of induction of inhalational general anesthesia is a function of the agent's blood/gas partition coefficient ($P_{b/g}$). Therefore:

1. The greater the $P_{b/g}$, the faster unconsciousness will be obtained.
2. Induction is slower with methoxyflurane than with isoflurane.
3. Induction is faster with halothane than with nitrous oxide.
4. The speed of induction is about the same with isoflurane and enflurane.

23–6 Characteristic signs of Stage III, Plane 2 of general anesthesia ("surgical anesthesia") are:

1. Subdued but regular breathing.
2. Constricted pupils.
3. Fixed eyeballs.
4. Rigid, tense muscles.

23–7 Nitrous oxide is used widely in anesthesia because it:

1. Is nonflammable and nonexplosive.
2. Provides rapid, smooth induction of anesthesia.
3. Produces excellent analgesia.
4. Is a potent muscle relaxant.

23–8 General anesthetic agents that sensitize the myocardium to exogenous catecholamines include:

1. Thiopental.
2. Isoflurane.
3. Enflurane.
4. Halothane.

23–9 The inhalational general anesthetics halothane and enflurane have which of the following characteristics in common?

1. They are respiratory depressants.
2. Hypotension and depression of the myocardium are dose-dependent.
3. They may precipitate malignant hyperthermia in genetically predisposed subjects.
4. About 20% of an inhaled dose of each agent is metabolized.

23–10 The ultrashort action of thiobarbiturates, as used in general anesthesia, is due to:

1. Rapid biotransformation.
2. High selectivity for brain tissue.
3. Strong binding to plasma proteins.
4. Rapid redistribution in body tissues.

24–1 Local anesthetics block:

1. Small neurons before large neurons.
2. Pain neurons before pressure neurons.
3. Demyelinated nerve terminals before myelinated nerve axons.
4. Inhibitory CNS neurons before excitatory CNS neurons.

24–2 Concerning local anesthetics:

1. Anesthesia occurs when a sufficiently high concentration has been achieved in the membrane, which is similar for all local anesthetics.
2. In the membrane the drugs are present in both the charged and the uncharged forms.
3. Anesthetic potency and anesthetic toxicity increase with lipid solubility.
4. In the membrane the outward movement of K^+ is affected more than the inward movement of Na^+.

24–3 The influence of pH on local anesthetic potency is an important consideration because:

1. Most local anesthetics are tertiary amines.
2. The uncharged form of the drug will readily permeate neuronal membranes.
3. The charged form produces most of the local anesthetic blockade.
4. Different sites of drug application have different pH.

24–4 Local anesthetic potency increases with:

1. Increasing lipid solubility.
2. Increasing hydrogen ion concentration.
3. Decreasing susceptibility to serum cholinesterase.
4. Increasing neuronal diameter.

24–5 Local anesthetics:

1. Are equipotent at a membrane concentration of 5000 μmol/100 mL membrane.
2. Expand membranes by interacting with membrane lipids and proteins.
3. Inhibit the inward flow of sodium ions.
4. Inhibit the electrotonic spread of membrane potentials.

24–6 Actions other than local anesthesia, variously caused by local anesthetics, include:

1. Local vasoconstriction.
2. Central nervous system stimulation.
3. Blockade of synaptic impulse transmission.
4. Decreased myocardial excitability.

24–7 The duration of action of local anesthetics may be increased:

1. By local coadministration of epinephrine [adrenaline].
2. In patients with a genetic deficiency of plasma cholinesterase.
3. By replacing an ester bond with an amide bond.
4. In patients with liver disease.

24–8 Concerning clinical uses of local anesthetics:

1. Cocaine is too toxic for other than topical use on the eye and the nasopharynx.
2. Procaine causes vasoconstriction at the site of application, which prolongs its local anesthetic action.
3. Tetracaine has about 10–15 times the anesthetic potency and systemic toxicity of procaine.
4. Lidocaine shows the highest degree of plasma protein binding and the longest duration of action.

25–1 Concerning the absorption and distribution of ethanol:

1. Gastrointestinal absorption is highest from beverages containing 20–30% ethanol.
2. The volume of distribution equals total body water.
3. Attainment of equilibrium concentrations between blood and various tissue fluids is a function of blood flow to different tissues.
4. The rate of loss in urine, breath, and sweat is proportional to the plasma concentration.

25–2 The *in vivo* metabolism of ethanol:

1. Can be described by pseudo-zero-order kinetics.
2. Occurs at an average rate of 10 g/hr.
3. Is controlled by the rate of NADH reoxidation.
4. Depends most importantly on the microsomal ethanol-oxidizing system.

25–3 Concerning the oxidation of ethanol:

1. Complete ethanol oxidation in the body yields about 7 cal/g.
2. The rate-limiting factor in the process is the acetaldehyde dehydrogenase step.
3. The rate of ethanol oxidation is increased in chronic heavy drinkers.
4. The NAD concentration or NAD : NADH ratio determines the rate of oxidation in normal individuals.

25–4 Blood ethanol levels can be determined by breath analysis because:

1. The ethanol concentrations in the alveolar air and the brain are the same.
2. The ethanol concentration in alveolar air equals that of plasma.
3. The blood/air partition coefficient is the same as the blood/brain partition coefficient.
4. Blood ethanol is in rapid equilibrium with the alveolar air.

25–5 Concerning metabolic and endocrine effects of ethanol:

1. Elevation of serum lactate may precipitate attacks of gout.
2. Rising blood ethanol levels inhibit secretion of pituitary antidiuretic hormone.
3. Large intakes of ethanol may cause hypoglycemia due to decreased gluconeogenesis.
4. Intoxicating doses of ethanol tend to lower plasma corticosteroid and catecholamine levels.

25–6 Behavioral effects of ethanol:

1. Correlate closely with blood alcohol levels.
2. Can be potentiated by numerous other CNS-active drugs.
3. Are the result of stimulation of the reticular activating system.
4. Are influenced by factors in the environmental setting.

25–7 Ethanol:

1. Can initiate compensatory changes that give rise to acute tolerance.
2. Can protect individuals against the effects of cold exposure by preventing heat loss.
3. Acts as an antidote for methanol poisoning in humans.
4. Inhibits gastric acid secretion and motility of the GI tract.

25–8 Alcohol-dependent individuals:

1. Can tolerate larger doses of ethanol because of faster oxidation in the liver.
2. Require larger doses of general anesthetics because of nervous system cross-tolerance.
3. Show a maximum degree of tolerance to ethanol that is much smaller than the tolerance to opiates or benzodiazepines.
4. Must consume larger amounts of ethanol because of chronic polyuria.

25–9 Symptoms of ethanol withdrawal after prolonged periods of heavy alcohol consumption include:

1. Hyperirritability.
2. Tremor.
3. Sweating.
4. Sleeplessness.

25–10 Disulfiram (tetra-ethyl thiuram disulfide):

1. Is an effective treatment of alcohol withdrawal syndromes.
2. Prevents oxidation of acetaldehyde to acetate.
3. Protects the liver against damage by alcohol.
4. Impairs synthesis of catecholamines in nerve endings.

26–1 Benzodiazepine receptors:

1. Are highest in density in the cerebral cortex.
2. Are functionally linked to postsynaptic GABA receptors.
3. Are thought to regulate chloride conductance in the presence of GABA.
4. Can be blocked experimentally by Ro 15-1788 (new name flumazenil).

26–2 Concerning the pharmacokinetics of benzodiazepines:

1. Most benzodiazepines are not significantly bound to serum proteins.
2. All benzodiazepines are biotransformed in the liver, some to active metabolites.
3. Volumes of distribution of individual drugs are inversely proportional to their lipid solubility.
4. Metabolic desmethyl derivatives significantly extend the durations of action of parent compounds.

26–3 Therapeutic indications for benzodiazepines include:

1. Acute anxiety disorders.
2. Some types of epilepsy.
3. Abnormally high skeletal muscle tone.
4. Psychotic states.

26–4 Benzodiazepines:

1. Can give rise to tolerance and physical dependence.
2. Interact with many other psychoactive drugs.
3. Have adverse effects that are direct extensions of their pharmacologic actions.
4. In overdose have a very wide safety margin.

26–5 Pentobarbital differs significantly from phenobarbital in that it is:

1. Longer acting.
2. Faster acting.
3. Less likely to be abused.
4. More likely to cause physical dependence and withdrawal symptoms.

26–6 Clinical uses of barbiturates include:

1. Some types of epilepsy.
2. Chronic anxiety disorders.
3. Induction of general anesthesia.
4. Intractable cancer pain.

26–7 Undesirable or toxic effects of barbiturates include:

1. Respiratory depression.
2. Precipitation of attacks of porphyria.
3. Tolerance and addiction.
4. Tachycardia and hypertension.

26–8 Advantages of benzodiazepines over barbiturates as sedative-hypnotics are:

1. Less drowsiness.
2. Fewer drug interactions.
3. Fewer or no withdrawal symptoms.
4. Less likely to be suicidally effective.

27–1 Concerning the mechanisms of action of neuroleptics:

1. They act selectively on dopamine receptors.
2. Drug molecules can adopt a certain shape or conformation that is similar to dopamine.
3. The dopamine receptor blockade is competitive.
4. Neuroleptics also block the actions of exogenous dopamine receptor agonists.

27–2 The enzymes involved in neuronal dopamine synthesis and breakdown include:

1. Tyrosine hydroxylase.
2. Dopa decarboxylase.
3. Monoamine oxidase.
4. Catechol-O-methyl transferase.

27–3 Concerning dopamine receptors:

1. They exist as D_1 and D_2 types.
2. The D_1 type exists in a high-affinity and a low-affinity state.
3. Neuroleptics block D_2 receptors, causing disinhibition of neurons.
4. Receptor blockade results in feedback inhibition of dopamine synthesis.

27–4 Chlorpromazine:

1. Reduces the activity in the ascending reticular formation.
2. Depresses hypothalamic functions.
3. Depresses the arousal response in the limbic system.
4. Reduces the nausea of motion sickness.

27–5 Adverse effects of neuroleptics include:

1. Drug-induced nephropathy.
2. Acute dyskinesias and dystonias.
3. Acute hypertensive crises.
4. Drug-induced akathisia.

27–6 Neuroleptic-induced extrapyramidal signs include:

1. Restriction of body motions.
2. Stiffness and rigidity.
3. Tremor.
4. Epileptiform seizures.

27–7 Tardive dyskinesia, which is sometimes seen in long-term neuroleptic therapy:

1. Occurs when a supersensitive state causes predominance of dopaminergic input.
2. Consists of movement disorders that are indistinguishable from parkinsonism.
3. May be managed by withholding the neuroleptic, thus facilitating recovery.
4. Can be moderated by adding an anticholinergic drug to the treatment regimen.

27–8 Neuroleptics are primarily used to treat:

1. Major affective disorders.
2. Schizophrenias.
3. Epilepsies.
4. Organic psychoses.

27–9 Neuroleptics of the phenothiazine type include:

1. Chlorpromazine.
2. Pimozide.
3. Thioridazine.
4. Haloperidol.

27–10 Pseudopregnancy:

1. Is a constellation of symptoms such as absence of menstruation, hyperprolactinemia, swollen breasts, and galactorrhea.
2. Is caused in part by neuroleptic blockade of dopamine receptors on mammotroph cells of the hypothalamus.
3. Is caused in part by neuroleptic blockade of FSH and LH release.
4. As a side effect of neuroleptic therapy has no analogous symptomatology in men.

28–1 Which of the following centrally acting drugs belong to the group of tricyclic antidepressants?

1. Tranylcypromine.
2. Doxepin.
3. Chlorpromazine.
4. Amitriptyline.

28–2 Mechanisms by which tricyclic antidepressants are believed to act on mood and behavior include:

1. Down-regulation of postsynaptic β adrenoceptors.
2. Blockade of norepinephrine [noradrenaline] re-uptake.
3. Inhibition of serotonin re-uptake.
4. Blockade of dopamine re-uptake.

28–3 Tricyclic antidepressants:

1. Are generally well absorbed from the gastrointestinal tract.
2. Have half-lives that increase with the duration of therapy.
3. Require several days or weeks for full therapeutic effect.
4. Can have active metabolites depending on the molecular structure of the parent drug.

28–4 Common adverse effects of tricyclic antidepressants include:

1. Dryness of the mouth.
2. Drowsiness and faulty memory.
3. Postural hypotension.
4. Urinary retention and constipation.

28–5 Tricyclic antidepressants should be used cautiously or not at all in patients receiving:

1. Monoamine oxidase inhibitors.
2. Sympathomimetics.
3. Anticonvulsants.
4. Anxiolytics.

28–6 During treatment of a depressed patient with monoamine oxidase inhibitors:

1. The patient must avoid certain cheeses, wines, and yeast products.
2. The drugs are taken at bedtime because of their sedative action.
3. There may be a noticeable increase in appetite and body weight.
4. There is a preponderance of parasympathetic over sympathetic side effects.

28–7 Side effects of monoamine oxidase inhibitors:

1. Are in many respects similar to those of tricyclic antidepressants.
2. Can be minimized with β-blocker therapy.
3. In overdose resemble those of amphetamine overdosage.
4. Terminate quickly upon withdrawal of the offending drug.

28–8 Lithium:

1. Produces neither depressant nor euphoriant effects in normal individuals.
2. Is rapidly absorbed from the gastrointestinal tract, but attainment of full therapeutic effects requires 2–3 weeks.
3. Excretion will be impaired, with the risk of intoxication, in patients on sodium-restricted diet or diuretics.
4. Has no significant side effects if serum levels are maintained within the therapeutic range.

29–1 Lysergic acid diethylamide (LSD):

1. Is readily and completely absorbed from the gastrointestinal tract.
2. Has a very long half-life because of strong plasma protein binding.
3. Acts primarily on 5-HT receptors and secondarily on dopamine receptors.
4. Does not produce tolerance even when taken at short intervals.

29–2 Concerning the LSD syndrome:

1. Somatic symptoms are the effects of strong central sympathomimetic stimulation.
2. Perceptual symptoms are of a predominantly visual-optical nature.
3. Emotional reactions are strongly influenced by the user's mood, the setting, and the presence of other people.
4. The most common ill effects are psychological, such as serious psychotic breakdown or spontaneous "flashbacks."

29–3 Amphetamines:

1. Are chemically related to norepinephrine [noradrenaline], ephedrine, and mescaline.
2. Have systemic physiologic and psychological effects that are almost identical to those of cocaine.
3. In high doses can produce acute psychosis with auditory hallucinations, stereotyped behavior, and paranoid delusions.
4. Produce psychic dependence and tolerance regardless of specific use and method of administration.

29–4 Concerning medical uses of amphetamines:

1. When used to enhance performance, the drugs will also diminish the awareness of fatigue.
2. The drugs are frequently prescribed for their anorexic effect because this use carries none of the usual risks.
3. Hyperkinetic children show paradoxical sedation with amphetamines, which permits empiric management of this disorder.
4. Large doses are used for their analeptic effects to hasten recovery from general anesthesia.

29–5 The main features of the atropine syndrome are:

1. Confusion, disorientation, and memory loss.
2. Tactile, auditory, and visual hallucinations.
3. Hyperthermia and hyperreflexia.
4. Typically brief duration with no residual effects.

29–6 The main medical and social uses of cocaine are:

1. As an anesthetic for infiltrative, regional, and spinal anesthesia.
2. As a psychotomimetic to be sniffed for absorption by the nasal mucosa.
3. As an anorexic administered orally to promote weight loss.
4. As a hallucinogen when inhaled as the free base for rapid absorption into the pulmonary circulation.

29–7 Phencyclidine (PCP):

1. Produces a mental state similar to that caused by atropine.
2. Has peripheral antimuscarinic effects that are the same as those of atropine.
3. Has analgesic and anesthetic properties.
4. Together with ketamine belongs to the drugs used in clinical "dissociative" anesthesia.

29–8 Tetrahydrocannabinol (THC):

1. Is not absorbed by any route other than inhalation of marijuana smoke.
2. Is rapidly inactivated by conversion to 11-hydroxy-THC.
3. Produces cross-tolerance to LSD- and amphetamine-like drugs.
4. Has an elimination half-life of about 56 hours in humans.

29–9 The smoking of cannabis produces:

1. Tachycardia, conjunctival reddening, EEG slowing, mild euphoria, and driving impairment (acute effects, low to moderate doses).
2. Distortions of space and time perception, reverie-like hallucinations, and acute psychoses (acute effects, high doses).
3. Chronic bronchitis and premalignant changes in bronchial epithelium (chronic daily use, high doses).
4. Synergism with both amphetamine and barbiturates in different stages of acute intoxication.

AUTACOIDS AND MEDIATORS/MODIFIERS OF TISSUE RESPONSES

30–1 Concerning eicosanoids:

1. They are oxygenation products derived from phospholipids by the action of phospholipase A_2.
2. The lipoxygenase pathway results in the formation of leukotrienes.
3. Prostaglandins are products derived from the cyclooxygenase pathway.
4. The epoxygenase pathway is catalyzed by a cytochrome P-450 monooxygenase system.

30–2 Cyclic endoperoxides (PGG_2 and PGH_2) are the immediate precursors of:

1. Prostaglandins D_2, E_2, $F_{2\alpha}$.
2. Prostacyclin PGI_2.
3. Thromboxane A_2.
4. Lipoxins A_3, B_3.

30–3 15-Hydroxy-prostaglandin dehydrogenase is the primary enzyme responsible for the rapid inactivation of:

1. Thromboxane A_2.
2. Prostaglandin I_2.
3. Leukotriene A_4.
4. Prostaglandin E_2.

30–4 Stages of the arachidonic acid cascade that can be influenced by drugs include:

1. Inhibition of cyclooxygenase by nonsteroidal anti-inflammatory agents.
2. Inactivation of thromboxane synthetase by corticosteroids.
3. Inhibition of prostacyclin synthetase by tranylcypromine.
4. Inactivation of prostaglandin endoperoxide isomerase by eicosatetraynoic acid.

30–5 Human *in vivo* effects of the eicosanoids include:

1. Vasoconstriction by thromboxane A_2.
2. Bronchial muscular relaxation by prostaglandin E_2.
3. Uterine muscular contraction by prostaglandin $F_{2\alpha}$.
4. Stimulation of gastric acid secretion by prostaglandin D_2.

30–6 The biologic activities of leukotrienes consist of:

1. Coronary vasodilatation.
2. Increased vascular wall permeability.
3. Bronchial and bronchiolar dilatation.
4. Mediation of some immediate hypersensitivity responses.

31–1 The enzymes involved in angiotensin generation include:

1. Renin.
2. Peptidyl dipeptidase.
3. Aminopeptidase.
4. Kininase I.

31–2 Induction of renin release from the kidneys normally results in:

1. Increased systemic blood pressure.
2. Vagus-mediated bradycardia.
3. Retention of sodium.
4. Promotion of diuresis.

31–3 Captopril and related drugs:

1. Are competitive inhibitors of peptidyl dipeptidase.
2. Are clinical antihypertensive agents.
3. Cause accumulation of kinins in most vascular beds.
4. Indirectly reduce the release of aldosterone from the adrenal cortex.

31–4 Aprotinin:

1. Belongs to the class of angiotensin converting enzyme (ACE) inhibitors.
2. Blocks the action of kininase II.
3. Promotes the breakdown of bradykinin.
4. Is used in the therapy of some hyperproteolytic states.

31–5 The enzymes responsible for the biosynthesis and metabolism of 5-hydroxytryptamine (5-HT, serotonin) are:

1. Tryptophan-5-hydroxylase.
2. Aromatic L-amino acid decarboxylase.
3. Monoamine oxidase.
4. Aldehyde dehydrogenase.

31–6 Endogenous serotonin:

1. Acts as a central inhibitory neurotransmitter.
2. Participates in the regulation of adenohypophysial secretions.
3. Is involved in the pathogenesis of migraine.
4. Is found in highest concentration in the brain, with small amounts in platelets.

31–7 Clinically useful drugs that influence endogenous serotonin include:

1. Lysergic acid, which antagonizes many peripheral actions of 5-HT.
2. Morphine, which blocks 5-HT action on the intestine.
3. Methysergide, which terminates acute migraine attacks by direct 5-HT receptor antagonism.
4. Pizotyline, which as a prophylactic reduces the frequency or severity of migraine attacks.

32–1 Histamine:

1. Is formed chiefly in the lungs, skin, and gastrointestinal mucosa by decarboxylation of histidine.
2. Is released from tissues after cell damage, and by substances that act as histamine liberators.
3. Effects are mediated through receptors that are designated H_1 and H_2.
4. Is inactivated by N-methylation (N-methyltransferase) or oxidative deamination (histaminase).

32–2 Pharmacologic effects of histamine include:

1. The classical "triple response" to local skin injury (H_1 and H_2 receptors).
2. Smooth muscle stimulation in bronchioles and intestine (H_1 receptors).
3. Reduced peripheral vascular resistance (H_1 and H_2 receptors).
4. Stimulation of gastric HCl secretion (H_2 receptors).

32–3 So-called conventional antihistamines (H_1-receptor blockers):

1. All have a similar basic structure that resembles that of histamine itself.
2. Antagonize all the actions of histamine by competitive receptor blockade.
3. Are distributed in all tissues, including the central nervous system.
4. Are all equally effective against motion sickness by paralyzing the vomiting control center.

32–4 Antihistaminic drugs produce a variety of side effects, including:

1. Sedation and CNS depression.
2. Local anesthesia.
3. Anticholinergic activity.
4. Anorexia and weight loss.

32–5 In accordance with selectively predominant activity, H_1-receptor blockers are used therapeutically:

1. To suppress allergic phenomena such as hay fever, urticaria, and serum sickness.
2. To raise the seizure threshold in epilepsy.
3. To suppress vestibular- and chemoreceptor-mediated emesis.
4. To terminate acute asthmatic attacks.

32–6 Histamine H_2-receptor blockers in current use:

1. Have very little, if any, affinity for H_1 receptors.
2. Inhibit gastric acid secretion induced by histamine, gastrin, or pentagastrin.
3. Are used to treat acute duodenal and benign gastric ulcers, gastroesophageal reflux, and gastric hypersecretory states.
4. Are considered to be practically nontoxic when used in clinically effective doses.

33–1 Salicylates such as acetylsalicylic acid (ASA, aspirin):

1. Provide analgesia by acting on central subcortical sites as well as on peripheral chemoreceptors.
2. Lower elevated body temperature by direct action on hypothalamic thermoregulatory centers.
3. Have anti-inflammatory activity that is due in part to inhibition of prostaglandin synthesis.
4. Reduce uric acid concentrations in the blood but are without effect on urate crystal deposits in joints and tissues.

33–2 Acetylsalicylic acid (ASA, aspirin) in toxic doses may cause:

1. Hyperventilation and respiratory alkalosis.
2. Respiratory and metabolic acidosis.
3. Delirium, convulsions, and coma.
4. Death from respiratory failure.

33–3 Long-term or inappropriate use of salicylates may give rise to:

1. Analgesic-induced nephropathy, most often in elderly women with histories of peptic ulcer, headaches, and arthralgias.
2. Bone marrow depression with aplastic anemia, agranulocytosis, and thrombocytopenia.
3. Reye's syndrome in young children during indiscriminate use of antipyretics in the course of some viral infections.
4. Increased incidence of coronary thrombosis and myocardial infarction in elderly men and heavy smokers.

33–4 Concerning the pharmacokinetics of acetylsalicylic acid (ASA, aspirin):

1. Absorption of therapeutic doses is about 90% complete and occurs in both the stomach and the small intestine.
2. The plasma half-life is about 15 minutes because of rapid renal excretion of the unchanged drug.
3. Salicylates bind to serum albumin, with potential displacement of other acidic drugs from protein binding sites.
4. The drug does not cross the blood-brain barrier and the placenta, and it is not secreted in breast milk.

33–5 Acetaminophen:

1. Is a chemical analog of acetylsalicylic acid with a spectrum of effects very similar to those of ASA.
2. Is largely inactivated by conjugation with glucuronic, sulfuric, and mercapturic acids.
3. Is a nontoxic alternative drug to ASA in the treatment of rheumatoid arthritis.
4. In ordinary doses causes virtually no side effects or drug interactions.

33–6 Phenylbutazone:

1. Belongs to the class of pyrazolone anti-inflammatory agents.
2. Has a mechanism of action based on inhibition of prostaglandin synthesis and stabilization of lysosomal membranes.
3. Undergoes hepatic biotransformation to two active metabolites.
4. Has uricosuric effects due to inhibition of tubular reabsorption of uric acid by one of its metabolites.

33–7 Indomethacin:

1. Is a very potent uricosuric agent that cannot be used for any other purpose.
2. Requires *in vivo* transformation to its pharmacologically active form.
3. Has weak anti-inflammatory activity through one of its metabolites.
4. Causes a variety of adverse effects that affect primarily the gastrointestinal tract.

33–8 The group of phenylpropionic acid derivatives:

1. Includes the drugs ibuprofen, fenoprofen, ketoprofen, flurbiprofen, naproxen, and tiaprofenic acid.
2. Is of value in the treatment of rheumatic disorders and other inflammatory conditions, as well as in the control of pain of varied origin.
3. Has a spectrum of adverse effects that are qualitatively similar to those of acetylsalicylic acid.
4. Lacks the toxic property of acetylsalicylic acid to cause gastric ulceration and bleeding.

33–9 Which of the following analgesic drugs can safely be administered to patients who cannot tolerate acetylsalicylic acid because of recurrent gastric ulcer problems?

1. Tiaprofenic acid.
2. Phenylbutazone.
3. Mefenamic acid.
4. Acetaminophen.

33–10 Gold compounds:

1. Are injected into rheumatic joints for the acute relief of severely debilitating pain.
2. Should be used only in rapidly progressive rheumatoid arthritis that responded poorly to conventional therapy.
3. Are believed to exert a local anesthetic effect on joint surfaces.
4. When absorbed may cause numerous side effects such as dermatitis, renal tubular damage, blood dyscrasias, encephalitis.

33–11 Properties of colchicine that are utilized in the treatment of acute gouty arthritis include:

1. Dissolution of uric acid crystals.
2. Inhibition of histamine release.
3. Arrest of cell division in metaphase.
4. Prevention of granulocyte and leukocyte mobilization.

33–12 Allopurinol:

1. Reduces plasma uric acid concentration by inhibition of xanthine oxidase.
2. Is not effective in hyperuricemia caused by other drugs, such as some diuretics.
3. Prevents the development or progression of chronic gouty arthritis.
4. Is excreted in unchanged form by renal glomerular filtration and tubular secretion.

CARDIOVASCULAR SYSTEM

34–1 Digitalis preparations in current clinical use are glycosides derived from:

1. *Digitalis purpurea.*
2. *Strophanthus hispidus.*
3. *Digitalis lanata.*
4. *Urginea maritima.*

34–2 Concerning the structure of digitalis glycosides:

1. Digoxin differs from digitoxin in that it has an -OH group at the C-12 position of the steroid nucleus.
2. The steroid nucleus and the lactone ring at the C-17 position together are called an "aglycone."
3. The aglycone moiety elicits the cardiotonic effects of the glycosides.
4. The steroid nucleus and the sugar residue at the C-3 oxygen together are called a "genin."

34–3 The positive inotropic effects of cardiac glycosides are the result of:

1. β_1-Adrenoceptor stimulation, raising intracellular cAMP.
2. Partial inhibition of sarcolemmal (Na^+ + K^+) -ATPase.
3. Activation of protein kinase C and phosphorylation of proteins.
4. Increased entry of Ca^{2+} into myocardial cells.

34–4 Electrophysiologic effects of digitalis glycosides include:

1. Dose-dependent increase in automaticity in all cardiac tissues.
2. Decreased conduction velocity in the A-V node and Purkinje system.
3. Increased effective refractory period of the A-V node.
4. Dose-dependent increase in vagal activity.

34–5 Extracardiac hemodynamic effects of digitalis glycosides are:

1. Increased sensitivity of carotid sinus baroreceptors.
2. Reduced systemic arteriolar resistance.
3. Increased renal blood flow and volume of glomerular filtrate.
4. Venous pooling of blood.

34–6 Digoxin:

1. In tablet form is 60–80% absorbed from the gastrointestinal tract.
2. Has an average half-life of 36 hours.
3. Is excreted principally unchanged in the urine.
4. Clearance is almost linearly related to creatinine clearance.

34–7 Digitoxin:

1. Absorption is low and unreliable; bioavailability is poor.
2. Is more strongly bound to plasma albumin than digoxin.
3. Has an average half-life of 4–6 hours.
4. Undergoes hepatic biotransformation followed by renal excretion.

34–8 Concerning digitalis toxicity:

1. Hypothyroid patients are particularly prone to develop toxicity.
2. Corticosteroids and thiazide diuretics tend to enhance toxicity.
3. Impaired renal function may cause an increase in digoxin half-life.
4. Toxicity is potentiated in the presence of low plasma sodium levels.

34–9 Manifestations of digitalis toxicity include:

1. Progressively more severe dysrhythmia.
2. Vomiting caused by stimulation of the chemoreceptor trigger zone.
3. A variety of visual disturbances.
4. Cumulation of potassium in myocardial cells.

34–10 Because of the low therapeutic index, individual digitalis dosage would depend very much on the patient's:

1. Hepatic and renal functions.
2. Plasma sodium levels.
3. Concomitant use of other drugs, such as quinidine, verapamil, and amiodarone.
4. Regularity of bowel movements.

35–1 Concerning the cardiac action potential:

1. In the resting state the transmembrane potential difference is maintained at −80 to −90 mV (inside vs. outside).
2. Excitation causes a rapid inward current of Na^+, which results in a steep upstroke of depolarization toward 0 mV (= phase 0).
3. Repolarization occurs during the slow inward movement of Ca^{2+} (= plateau), and the slow outward movement of K^+.
4. Spontaneous depolarization of pacemaker cells (*i.e.*, automaticity) is largely caused by a slow influx of Ca^{2+}.

35–2 Concerning the refractory period of myocardial cells:

1. The absolute refractory period is the time following initial depolarization in which the cell will not respond to any stimuli.
2. The relative refractory period contains the latter part of repolarization, during which stronger than normal stimuli can cause depolarization.
3. The effective refractory period is the shortest interval between two stimuli of equal strength that permits a propagated response.
4. Asynchrony of repolarization of myocardial cells (*i.e.*, conflicting refractory periods between cell groups) may render the heart vulnerable to the induction of arrhythmias.

35–3 The reentry phenomenon:

1. Is the short-circuiting of conducting tissue, causing a premature ventricular contraction.
2. Describes the entry of Na^{+} during depolarization of myocardial cell membranes.
3. Will cause sustained ventricular arrhythmia if it becomes repetitive.
4. Depends for its development on abnormal Ca^{2+} fluxes during repolarization of myocardial cell membranes.

35–4 The duration of the action potential in myocardial cells is prolonged by:

1. Amiodarone.
2. Bretylium.
3. Sotalol.
4. Lidocaine.

35–5 Which of the following antiarrhythmic drugs undergo transformation to active metabolites?

1. Encainide.
2. Bretylium.
3. Procainamide.
4. Sotalol.

35–6 The Q-T interval in the electrocardiogram is generally shortened by:

1. Quinidine.
2. Lidocaine.
3. Procainamide.
4. Phenytoin.

35–7 Quinidine

1. Decreases the slope of phase 4 spontaneous depolarization.
2. Prolongs the effective refractory period.
3. Suppresses normal automaticity.
4. Has a significant positive inotropic effect.

35–8 Procainamide:

1. Is similar to quinidine in its antiarrhythmic effects.
2. Has a relatively long half-life of about 12 hours.
3. May cause a syndrome resembling systemic lupus erythematosus.
4. May produce a hypertensive crisis when injected intravenously.

35–9 Lidocaine:

1. Is subject to significant first-pass transformation when given orally.
2. Is dealkylated to two metabolites, both of which are very active.
3. May cause convulsions and respiratory arrest in overdose.
4. Prolongs the effective refractory period.

35–10 Amiodarone:

1. Has a half-life of up to 60 days after long-term administration.
2. Has complex antiarrhythmic effects, dominated by prolongation of action potential duration and refractoriness.
3. Is a peripheral vasodilator and an effective antianginal agent.
4. Displays a wide spectrum of toxic effects, most often corneal microdeposits and, most dangerously, pulmonary fibrosis.

36–1 Vasodilators with action mainly or exclusively on arteriolar smooth muscle include:

1. Diazoxide.
2. Sodium nitroprusside.
3. Hydralazine.
4. Nitroglycerin.

36–2 Drugs that cause vasodilatation through a direct action on vascular smooth muscle include:

1. Diazoxide.
2. Hydralazine.
3. Minoxidil.
4. Prazosin.

36–3 Hemodynamic (indirect) effects of arterial vasodilators consist of increased:

1. Heart rate.
2. Venous return.
3. Myocardial oxygen consumption.
4. Myocardial force of contraction.

36–4 Hydralazine is known to:

1. Be subject to first-pass effects in the intestinal wall and liver.
2. Be biotransformed mainly by acetylation.
3. Cause systemic lupus erythematosus, primarily in slow acetylators.
4. Produce glucose intolerance and hyperglycemia.

36–5 Diazoxide and sodium nitroprusside *both:*

1. Are combined arterial and venous vasodilators.
2. Are administered intravenously.
3. Have prolonged hypotensive effects.
4. Are suitable in the treatment of hypertensive emergencies.

36–6 Nitroglycerin:

1. Diminishes venous return to the heart.
2. Rapidly reduces myocardial oxygen demand.
3. Tachycardia is the result of increased sympathetic discharge.
4. May produce "nitrite headache," to which tolerance develops.

36–7 Concerning sublingual administration of nitroglycerin:

1. It may be given to patients who already receive β blockers.
2. The onset of action is within 1–2 minutes.
3. Elimination is predominantly *via* hepatic biotransformation.
4. The duration of action is in excess of 1 hour.

36–8 Currently used calcium-channel blockers as a group of vasoactive drugs:

1. Are predominantly dilators of arterioles.
2. On an equimolar basis are equally active antihypertensives.
3. Are effective antianginal drugs.
4. Block specifically the phosphorylation-dependent gates in sarcolemmal membranes.

36–9 Nifedipine in therapeutic dosage causes a marked decrease in:

1. Systemic vascular resistance.
2. Heart rate.
3. Mean arterial pressure.
4. Cardiac output.

36–10 Verapamil in therapeutic dosage causes a marked decrease in:

1. Systemic vascular resistance.
2. Heart rate.
3. Mean arterial pressure.
4. Cardiac output.

37–1 Concerning lipoprotein transport:

1. Plasma cholesterol is carried predominantly by very-low-density lipoprotein (VLDL) and low-density lipoprotein (LDL).
2. VLDL is secreted from the liver and contains more cholesterol and less triglyceride than do chylomicrons.
3. Intermediate-density lipoprotein (IDL) and LDL provide cholesterol for the synthesis of cell membranes.
4. High-density lipoprotein (HDL) absorbs free cholesterol, which is then esterified before forming new VLDL and LDL.

37–2 Concerning lipoprotein pathophysiology:

1. HDL-cholesterol levels are always higher in adult males than in adult females.
2. In normal males, HDL-cholesterol levels decline during the first decades of life.
3. In females, plasma triglyceride levels rise steadily with increasing age, peaking at about age 40.
4. An increase in LDL:HDL ratio increases the risk of cardiovascular disease.

37–3 Which of the following hyperlipoproteinemia varieties are associated with increased risk of heart disease?

1. Primary endogenous hypertriglyceridemia.
2. Familial hypercholesterolemia.
3. Familial hyperlipidemia.
4. Familial hyperalphalipoproteinemia.

37–4 Lovastatin [mevinolin]:

1. Is a competitive inhibitor of HMg-CoA reductase.
2. Can lower plasma cholesterol by up to 40%.
3. Reduces plasma LDL by increasing the number of hepatic LDL receptors.
4. Reduces plasma LDL, HDL, and VLDL at similar rates.

37-5 Cholestyramine and colestipol:

1. Are bile-acid–binding resins.
2. Lower plasma LDL-cholesterol levels quickly within days.
3. Increase the number of LDL receptors with consequent increase in plasma clearance of LDL.
4. Commonly cause nausea, ototoxicity, and nephrotoxicity.

37–6 Clofibrate and gemfibrozil:

1. Impair conversion of plasma lipoproteins.
2. Increase lipoprotein lipase activity.
3. Lower plasma VLDL levels.
4. Are contraindicated in the presence of renal and hepatic impairment and in pregnancy.

38–1 Antihypertensive drug therapy:

1. Is used to counter pathophysiologic mechanisms that maintain high peripheral resistance and arteriolar tone.
2. Has caused a major reduction in death from myocardial infarction worldwide.
3. Has resulted in an overall reduction in morbidity and mortality from cerebrovascular strokes, congestive heart failure, and renal failure.
4. Is ineffective in "essential" hypertension of unknown etiology.

38–2 Diuretics:

1. As monotherapy are effective in mild to moderate hypertension.
2. Reduce extracellular fluid volume and circulating plasma volume and thus decrease venous return and cardiac output.
3. Cause long-term pressure reduction by lowering total peripheral vascular resistance.
4. Can enhance the hypotensive effects of other drugs.

38–3 Hydralazine:

1. Is a direct-acting vasodilator.
2. Causes reflex tachycardia that can be reduced by addition of a β blocker.
3. Has little effect on veins and therefore does not cause orthostatic hypotension.
4. Causes hirsutism as its most annoying side effect.

38–4 Hypertensive emergencies can be treated effectively with intravenous:

1. Captopril.
2. Labetalol.
3. Minoxidil.
4. Sodium nitroprusside.

38–5 Concerning calcium antagonists:

1. All agents cause postural hypotension.
2. Verapamil has pronounced negative inotropic action.
3. Diltiazem causes reflex tachycardia.
4. Nifedipine has the greatest vasodilator effect.

38–6 α-Methyldopa:

1. Is a direct-acting vascular smooth muscle relaxant.
2. Causes rapid disappearance of norepinephrine [noradrenaline] from adrenergic nerve terminals.
3. Acts as a blocker of peripheral α adrenoceptors.
4. Is transformed into a false transmitter that stimulates central α_2 adrenoceptors.

38–7 β Blockers may be contraindicated in:

1. Congestive heart failure with bradycardia.
2. Ventricular tachycardia.
3. Bronchial asthma.
4. Thyrotoxicosis.

38–8 "Cardioselectivity" of β blockers implies:

1. A certain pharmacokinetic profile.
2. Specificity for cardiac β receptors only.
3. Combined blockade of α and β adrenoceptors.
4. Safer use than nonselective drugs in bronchial asthma.

RESPIRATORY, RENAL, AND BLOOD SYSTEMS

39–1 Bronchial asthma:

1. Is a condition of dyspnea due mainly to spasms of bronchial smooth muscle.
2. Is triggered by a variety of mechanisms, such as infection, allergy, exercise, or psychogenic factors.
3. Responds to bronchodilator drugs, such as sympathomimetics, anticholinergics, and methylxanthines.
4. In its most severe manifestation is also known as "anaphylaxis."

39–2 Chemical mediators of bronchoconstriction include:

1. Acetylcholine.
2. Bradykinin.
3. Histamine.
4. Prostaglandin $F_{2\alpha}$.

39–3 The pharmacologic effects of therapeutic doses of selective β_2-adrenoceptor agonists, in addition to bronchodilatation, include:

1. Marked tachycardia and arrhythmias.
2. Skeletal muscle tremors.
3. Hypertension.
4. Increased ciliary activity.

39–4 Potential advantages of albuterol [salbutamol] over isoproterenol in the treatment of bronchial asthma include:

1. Longer duration of action.
2. Reduced effects on β_1 adrenoceptors.
3. Less cardiac stimulation with equipotent doses.
4. A greater degree of bronchodilatation.

39–5 The bronchodilating effect of theophylline is believed to be related to:

1. Inhibition of phosphodiesterase and consequent increase in cAMP in bronchial smooth muscle.
2. Activation of adenylate cyclase and consequent increase in cAMP in bronchial smooth muscle.
3. Influences on bronchial smooth muscle Ca^{2+} concentrations.
4. Improved contractility of skeletal muscle of the diaphragm.

39–6 In addition to bronchodilatation, methylxanthines:

1. Have direct positive chronotropic and inotropic effects on the heart.
2. Stimulate the secretion of gastric acid and digestive enzymes.
3. Cause nervousness, tremor, and insomnia.
4. Are mild diuretics.

39–7 Cromolyn sodium [sodium cromoglycate] causes:

1. Bronchodilatation in acute asthmatic attacks.
2. Inhibition of mediator release from sensitized mast cells.
3. Blockade of histamine H_1 receptors.
4. Very few side effects because of specialized topical aerosol administration.

39–8 Possible actions of glucocorticoid drugs in the therapy of bronchial asthma include:

1. Reduction of tissue sensitivity to antigens.
2. Anti-inflammatory activity.
3. Increased responsiveness of β_2 adrenoceptors.
4. Decreased responsiveness of muscarinic cholinoceptors.

39–9 Which of the following are used as antitussives?

1. Codeine.
2. Hydrocodone.
3. Dextromethorphan.
4. Methadone.

39–10 Centrally acting respiratory stimulants of clinical usefulness include:

1. Nicotine.
2. Pentylenetetrazole.
3. Acetylsalicylic acid.
4. Doxapram.

40–1 Which of the following chief renal sites of action of diuretics are correct?

1. Loop diuretics: medullary ascending limb of Henle's loop.
2. Sulfonamide diuretics: cortical ascending limb of Henle's loop and distal convoluted tubules.
3. Carbonic anhydrase inhibitors: proximal tubules.
4. Potassium-sparing diuretics: collecting tubules and ducts.

40–2 Loop diuretics (e.g., furosemide, ethacrynic acid):

1. Inhibit active chloride reabsorption in Henle's loop.
2. Impair formation of dilute as well as maximally concentrated urine.
3. Produce major calciuresis that accompanies the increased sodium excretion.
4. Remain effective even when the glomerular filtration rate is minimal ($<$ 30 mL/min).

40–3 Adverse and toxic effects of loop diuretics include:

1. Hypokalemia.
2. Hyperuricemia.
3. Carbohydrate intolerance.
4. Visual disturbances.

40–4 Furosemide is a useful agent to treat:

1. Congestive heart failure.
2. Hypercalciuria.
3. Pulmonary edema.
4. Diabetes insipidus.

40–5 Sulfonamide diuretics (*e.g.*, hydrochlorothiazide):

1. Decrease the intravascular fluid volume.
2. Increase the urinary excretion of calcium.
3. Inhibit insulin release.
4. Impair urinary concentrating capacity.

40–6 Unwanted side effects of hydrochlorothiazide include:

1. Deafness.
2. Hyperglycemia.
3. Hyperkalemia.
4. Hyperuricemia.

40–7 The thiazide diuretics are useful agents to treat:

1. Congestive heart failure.
2. Essential hypertension.
3. Diabetes insipidus.
4. Ascites.

40–8 Inhibition of carbonic anhydrase by acetazolamide causes increased urinary losses of:

1. Sodium.
2. Potassium.
3. Bicarbonate.
4. Chloride.

40–9 Major adverse effects of spironolactone include:

1. Hyperglycemia.
2. Hyperuricemia.
3. Hypercalcemia.
4. Hyperkalemia.

40–10 Spironolactone, triamterene, and amiloride:

1. Are only mildly effective diuretics.
2. Impair distal Na^+/K^+ exchange.
3. Frequently cause gastrointestinal distress.
4. Are useful in patients with congestive heart failure.

40–11 Osmotic diuretics (e.g., mannitol, urea):

1. Are administered intravenously.
2. Prevent sodium reabsorption by dilution of the intraluminal sodium concentration.
3. Markedly increase the tubular fluid flow rate.
4. Can cause acute intravascular volume depletion.

40–12 Metabolic alkalosis is seen with the chronic use of:

1. Chlorthalidone.
2. Furosemide.
3. Hydrochlorothiazide.
4. Acetazolamide.

41–1 Concerning blood coagulation:

1. Activation of factors XII and XI are interconversions that do not require calcium ions for completion.
2. The generation of prothrombin activator (*i.e.,* thromboplastic activity) may be delayed in the absence of phospholipid.
3. The majority of hemophilic syndromes are caused by defects or deficiencies of plasma factors VIII or IX.
4. The coagulation process follows the same mechanisms, whether it be physiologic hemostasis or pathologic thrombosis.

41–2 Blood platelet aggregation:

1. Is the usual first step in physiologic hemostasis.
2. May be promoted by pathologic changes in endothelial surfaces.
3. May be prevented by administration of nonsteroidal anti-inflammatory drugs.
4. Defects may cause the prothrombin time to be prolonged.

41–3 Physiologic substances that act as specific stimuli for the platelet release reaction include:

1. Angiotensin II.
2. Clotting factor XIIa.
3. Prostaglandin I_2.
4. Thromboxane A_2.

41–4 The agents that inhibit platelet aggregation by mechanisms *other than* inhibition of platelet cyclooxygenase are:

1. Sulfinpyrazone.
2. Phenylbutazone.
3. Indomethacin.
4. Dipyridamole.

41–5 Heparin:

1. Is a natural product of animal tissue origin.
2. Is active both *in vivo* and *in vitro.*
3. Half-life increases with increasing dose.
4. Is excreted unchanged in the urine.

41–6 The action of heparin is characterized by:

1. Activation of plasma antithrombin III.
2. Inactivation of factors involved in the generation of thromboplastic activity.
3. Neutralization of tissue thromboplastin.
4. Enhancement of the electronegative charge of vascular endothelium.

41–7 Coumarin compounds:

1. Block the release of preformed clotting factors by the liver.
2. Have enhanced anticoagulant effects in vitamin K deficiency.
3. Have typically short half-lives of less than 6 hours.
4. Have anticoagulant effects only *in vivo.*

41–8 Warfarin:

1. Is a synthetic compound.
2. Inhibits hepatic synthesis of clotting factors II, VII, IX, and X.
3. Is highly protein-bound in plasma.
4. Is subject to numerous drug-drug interactions.

41–9 Protamine sulfate is the specific antidote to neutralize:

1. Acetylsalicylic acid (ASA, aspirin).
2. Warfarin.
3. Streptokinase.
4. Heparin.

41–10 Intravascular fibrinolysis:

1. Results from the action of plasmin, a natural plasma enzyme.
2. Occurs after oral administration of streptokinase.
3. Is produced by activation of plasminogen with tissue-type plasminogen activator.
4. With urokinase is confined to blood clots in renal vessels.

42–1 Iron:

1. Is required for optimal hemoglobin synthesis.
2. Deficiency will be accompanied by megaloblastosis.
3. Is the specific agent to treat microcytic, hypochromic anemia.
4. Intoxication is treated specifically with $CaNa_2EDTA$.

42–2 Absorption of iron from the gastrointestinal tract:

1. Is enhanced in the presence of iron deficiency.
2. Occurs more readily when iron is in the ferrous state.
3. Is accelerated during increased demands of erythropoiesis.
4. Requires the presence of gastric co-enzymes.

42–3 Circulating plasma protein-bound iron is in the form of:

1. Ferritin.
2. Hemochromatin.
3. Hemoglobin.
4. Transferrin.

42–4 Concerning therapy of iron-deficiency anemia:

1. Compounds for oral use are in the form of iron salts.
2. Oral therapy employs maximally tolerated doses over several months for restoration of depleted iron stores.
3. Intravenous therapy requires precise dosage calculations on the basis of hemoglobin deficit and the state of tissue iron stores.
4. Excessive, chronic administration of iron without iron deficiency may lead to hemochromatosis.

42–5 Folic acid:

1. Is required as cofactor for purine and pyrimidine synthesis, and for amino acid interconversions.
2. Must be synthesized from dietary para-aminobenzoic acid.
3. Undergoes various reduction steps to its biologically active form.
4. Deficiency will commonly cause aplastic anemia.

42–6 Vitamin B_{12} deficiency:

1. Develops early because of rapid depletion of vitamin B_{12} body stores.
2. May lead to systemic megaloblastosis.
3. Is almost always due to inadequate diet.
4. Is treatable with parenteral administration of cyanocobalamin.

42–7 Pernicious anemia:

1. Is an abnormality of vitamin B_{12} absorption.
2. Usually develops from lack of "gastric intrinsic factor of Castle."
3. Is hematologically similar to folic acid–deficiency anemia.
4. May cause neurologic deficits from damage to myelin.

ENDOCRINE SYSTEMS

43–1 Oxytocin and vasopressin:

1. Are small decapeptides.
2. Are synthesized and stored in the posterior pituitary.
3. Have widely different biologic half-lives.
4. Are often released together by the same stimulus.

43–2 Concerning the structures of oxytocin and vasopressin:

1. In both hormones, six of the amino acids form ring structures.
2. Opening of the rings abolishes hormonal activity in both.
3. Differences are in positions 3 and 8: vasopressin = Phe (3) and Arg (8); oxytocin = iLeu (3) and Leu (8).
4. Inactivation is primarily by proteolytic cleavage between positions 1 and 2 (Cys-Tyr).

43–3 Concerning the actions of vasopressin:

1. It has antidiuretic activity by facilitating the reabsorption of water by the collecting ducts of the kidneys.
2. It causes selective vasoconstriction, which excludes coronary and cerebral blood vessels.
3. It stimulates uterine muscle, causing short contractions in both the pregnant and nonpregnant uterus.
4. It promotes hemophilia-like hemorrhagic tendencies by destruction of plasma clotting factor VIII.

43–4 Desmopressin (DDAVP):

1. Has a longer half-life than vasopressin.
2. On equimolar basis has greater antidiuretic potency than vasopressin.
3. Is usually administered intranasally as an isotonic saline solution.
4. Is currently the drug of choice to treat diabetes insipidus.

43–5 Concerning the actions of oxytocin:

1. The most important physiologic function is the initiation of labor and delivery.
2. The hormone causes "milk letdown" through postpartum stimulation of milk alveoli and ducts.
3. The major vascular effects in humans are constriction of circular fibers of smooth muscles and hypertension.
4. One of its selective therapeutic uses is the control of uterine atony and bleeding during and after delivery.

43–6 Concerning ergot alkaloids:

1. These compounds are all derivatives of lysergic acid.
2. Ergotamine tartrate causes vasoconstriction and is used in the treatment of migraine headaches.
3. Bromocriptine is used to treat hyperprolactinemia and acromegaly.
4. Ergonovine maleate stimulates uterine contractions and is used to induce labor.

44–1 Thyroxine:

1. Is one of the two active agents produced by the thyroid gland.
2. Serves as a circulating reservoir for triiodothyronine.
3. And triiodothyronine differ structurally only by one atom of iodine.
4. Has 5–10 times the hormonal activity of triiodothyronine.

44–2 Graves' disease:

1. Is characterized by overproduction and high circulating levels of thyroid-stimulating hormone.
2. Appears to be the major cause of thyroid hyperactivity.
3. Is often accompanied by exophthalmos, which can be produced experimentally by administering thyroid hormone.
4. Is recognized as an autoimmune disease in which thyroid-stimulating immunoglobulins activate thyrotropin receptors.

44–3 In the treatment of hypothyroidism (myxedema), clinically effective agents are:

1. L-thyroxine.
2. D-thyroxine.
3. L-triiodothyronine.
4. Diiodotyrosine.

44–4 Pharmacologic approaches to the therapy of hyperthyroidism include:

1. Radioactive iodine.
2. Thiourea and thionamides.
3. Lugol's iodine, B.P.
4. β Blockers.

44–5 Propylthiouracil:

1. Is an effective agent in the treatment of hyperthyroidism.
2. Inhibits the activity of thyroglobulin peroxidase.
3. Reduces the levels of iodinated thyroglobulin stored in thyroid follicles.
4. Can lower the blood levels of thyroid-stimulating hormone.

44–6 Methimazole:

1. Acts by interfering with the synthesis of thyroid hormones.
2. Prevents the active transport of iodide ions into follicular cells.
3. In high doses elevates blood levels of thyroid-stimulating hormone.
4. Secondarily inhibits the release of thyroid hormones from the gland.

45–1 Gonadotropin-releasing hormone:

1. Is an octapeptide resembling oxytocin.
2. Originates in the hypothalamus.
3. Is secreted continuously with little fluctuation over time.
4. Stimulates the release of LH and FSH from the anterior pituitary.

45–2 Mestranol:

1. Is a conjugated estrogen found in urine.
2. Is not absorbed after oral administration.
3. Has anabolic activity that is inseparable from its androgenic action.
4. Is structurally and functionally related to ethinyl estradiol.

45–3 Oral contraceptives:

1. Are used cyclically (21 days on and 7 days off).
2. Are generally not recommended for women over 40 years of age.
3. Are contraindicated in women with a history of cerebrovascular disease.
4. Carry increased risks of cardiovascular side effects and morbidity in women who smoke tobacco.

45–4 Adverse effects associated with the use of oral contraceptives include:

1. Edema.
2. Headache.
3. Thrombophlebitis.
4. Osteoporosis.

45–5 The risk of endometrial carcinoma from the use of estrogens is effectively minimized by using:

1. An estradiol ester intramuscularly.
2. Premarin instead of ethinyl estradiol.
3. Ethinyl estradiol cyclically with mestranol.
4. The estrogen cyclically with norethindrone.

45–6 Diethylstilbestrol:

1. Is a synthetic estrogen.
2. Has a steroid nucleus like ethinyl estradiol.
3. May cause genital abnormalities in later life after exposure in utero.
4. Is currently used as a post-coital contraceptive.

45–7 Clomiphene and tamoxifen:

1. Are analogs of chlorotrianisene.
2. Are referred to as "antiestrogens."
3. Are nonsteroidal compounds with estrogenic activity.
4. Inhibit the secretion of pituitary gonadotropins.

45–8 Progesterone:

1. Is the natural hormone of the corpus luteum.
2. Is partially biotransformed in the liver.
3. Is poorly absorbed when taken orally.
4. May cause salt and water retention.

45–9 Under suitable conditions, androgens stimulate:

1. Secretion of FSH and ICSH by the adenohypophysis.
2. Protein synthesis in the prostate.
3. Renal excretion of calcium.
4. Protein synthesis in skeletal muscles.

45–10 Anabolic steroids:

1. Can be effective in the treatment of aplastic anemia.
2. Can inhibit skeletal growth in preadolescent males.
3. May have direct effects on the liver, including hepatic carcinoma.
4. Do not cause virilization because of their selectively anabolic actions.

46–1 Insulin:

1. Is a protein consisting of three interconnected chains of amino acids.
2. Has a molecular weight of about 6000.
3. Is packaged together with glucagon in secretory granules of the islets of Langerhans.
4. Of animal origin has biologic activity in humans.

46–2 Concerning various insulin forms and preparations:

1. Crystalline zinc insulin is the only insulin preparation suitable for the emergency treatment of diabetic coma.
2. Ultralente insulin and protamine zinc insulin control blood sugar with similar kinetics.
3. Pork and human insulin differ from each other by one amino acid in the B chain.
4. Sulfated insulin is used in patients with insulin resistance.

46–3 Human insulin preparations:

1. Are available as regular, lente, and isophane (NPH) insulin.
2. Are similar to insulin from bovine sources in causing allergic reactions.
3. Are produced by recombinant DNA technology or by chemical conversion of porcine to human insulin.
4. Have a duration of action that is markedly longer than insulin from animal sources.

46–4 Protamine zinc insulin (PZI) acts for an appreciably longer time than:

1. Crystalline zinc insulin.
2. Isophane (NPH) insulin.
3. Semilente insulin.
4. Lente insulin.

46–5 Lente insulin:

1. Is synonymous with neutral protamine Hagedorn insulin.
2. Is formed by treating zinc insulin with protamine.
3. Acts as rapidly as crystalline zinc insulin, but with longer duration.
4. Is a mixture of differently sized insulin crystals.

46–6 Concerning the use of insulin in diabetics:

1. Insulin is usually administered by subcutaneous injection.
2. Long-acting preparations help maintain a continuous supply of circulating insulin with a minimum of injections.
3. Allergic reactions to insulin most often result from contaminants in the preparations.
4. The principal therapeutic objective of insulin therapy is the prevention of ketoacidosis.

46–7 Undesired side effects of insulin encountered in chronic use by diabetics include:

1. Hypoglycemic reactions from missed meals or dosage variations.
2. Local subcutaneous lumpiness from frequent injections at the same site.
3. Visual disturbances due to osmotic changes in ocular fluids.
4. Intolerance to alcohol similar to disulfiram reactions.

46–8 Sulfonylureas:

1. Are derivatives of p-aminobenzene sulfonic acid (sulfanilamide).
2. Mimic the action of insulin at insulin receptors.
3. Stimulate the release of insulin from pancreatic β cells.
4. Are a useful alternative to insulin in insulin-resistant patients.

46–9 Oral hypoglycemics of the sulfonylurea group include:

1. Tolbutamide.
2. Chlorpropamide.
3. Glyburide.
4. Metformin.

46–10 Tolbutamide:

1. Is of particular value in treating type I ("juvenile") diabetes.
2. Acts chiefly by increasing glycolysis in tissue cells.
3. Decreases the incidence of cardiovascular complications of diabetes mellitus.
4. May cause hypoglycemic reactions in patients with mild diabetes.

47–1 Mineralocorticoid actions include:

1. Demineralization of bone.
2. Increased serum potassium levels.
3. Decreased renal tubular reabsorption of uric acid.
4. Increased serum sodium levels.

47–2 Glucocorticoid actions include:

1. Increased concentration of liver glycogen.
2. Reduced intensity of inflammatory responses.
3. Feedback inhibition of ACTH production.
4. Reduced production of gastric HCl and pepsin.

47–3 Cortisol (hydrocortisone):

1. Is one of the naturally occurring human adrenal corticosteroids.
2. Stimulates the secretion of adrenocorticotropic hormone.
3. Has toxic effects that are related to both glucocorticoid and mineralocorticoid activity.
4. As a natural hormone is not bound to plasma proteins.

47–4 Cortisol (hydrocortisone) may cause:

1. Nitrogen retention.
2. Sodium retention.
3. Potassium retention.
4. Fluid retention.

47–5 Glucocorticoids administered over prolonged periods may cause:

1. Changes in mood and behavior.
2. Increased susceptibility to infection.
3. Osteoporosis.
4. Adrenal insufficiency.

47–6 Prednisone:

1. Is converted to a more active product by hepatic biotransformation.
2. Has less mineralocorticoid activity than cortisol.
3. Opposes many of the metabolic effects of insulin.
4. Stimulates protein synthesis and accumulation in muscle tissue.

47–7 Prednisolone is suitable for single-steroid therapy of:

1. Primary adrenal cortical insufficiency (Addison's disease).
2. Bronchial asthma with allergic basis.
3. Cushing's syndrome.
4. Severe chronic eczema.

47–8 Dexamethasone:

1. Is a synthetic fluorinated corticosteroid.
2. Has much more glucocorticoid activity than cortisol.
3. Has much less mineralocorticoid activity than cortisone.
4. Is used in lower dosage than prednisone.

47–9 Which of the following drugs would be required for long-term hormonal replacement therapy in an adult male whose pituitary gland had been surgically removed?

1. Adrenocorticotropic hormone (ACTH).
2. Liothyronine.
3. Desmopressin (DDAVP).
4. Cortisone.

47–10 Metyrapone:

1. Inhibits 11-β-hydroxylase.
2. Indirectly increases the synthesis of 11-desoxycortisol.
3. Can be used diagnostically to test pituitary function.
4. Is used therapeutically to increase aldosterone production.

48–1 Calcium salts:

1. Are specific in the treatment of low calcium states.
2. Are used as dietary supplements in osteoporosis or osteomalacia.
3. Interfere with the oral absorption of tetracycline.
4. Administered in excess for long periods will cause tetany.

48–2 Fluoride:

1. Stimulates the synthesis of bone matrix by osteoblasts.
2. Accelerates the mineralization of newly formed bone matrix.
3. In municipal water supplies carries a low risk of toxicity because the concentration normally does not exceed 1 ppm.
4. Absorption from the gastrointestinal tract is enhanced by the co-administration of calcium.

48–3 Diphosphonates:

1. Inhibit the resorption and mineralization of bone.
2. Are used clinically in the treatment of Paget's disease of bone.
3. May decrease the risk of heterotopic ossification following total hip replacement.
4. Appear to be nontoxic when used in doses not exceeding 20 mg/kg/day for not more than 4 months.

49–1 Concerning vitamin consumption and vitamin toxicity:

1. The toxicity of a vitamin is directly proportional to the degree of its storage in tissues.
2. Toxicity is never seen with those vitamins which, if eaten in excess, can be secreted in the urine.
3. Excessive intakes of any one of the four fat-soluble vitamins consistently produce toxicity because the excess cannot be excreted in the urine.
4. Toxicity of a vitamin is more likely to occur from large intakes due to "therapeutic" dosing than from excessive intakes of specific foods.

49–2 Which of the following deficiency signs are characteristic for the vitamins listed?

1. Hemorrhagic lesions of the gums and skin: vitamin C.
2. Dermatitis, atrophy of the gastrointestinal mucosa, diarrhea, and mental confusion: niacin.
3. Polyneuropathy and muscle wasting: thiamin.
4. Decalcification of bone matrix and bone deformities: vitamin D.

49–3 Concerning the functions of vitamins:

1. The role of vitamin A in the visual process is related to the production of rhodopsin in the rod cells and of iodopsin in the cone cells of the retina.
2. The function and maintenance of peripheral nervous tissue are directly dependent on folic acid (folate) and its role in DNA synthesis.
3. Vitamins C and E are considered to be the major vitamins having antioxidant or free radical-scavenging activity in the tissues.
4. Interconversion of macronutrients and production of energy require the integrated function of enzyme systems in which all B vitamins have a direct role.

49–4 Concerning the role of vitamins in bone matrix and collagen formation and in calcification of bone:

1. Vitamin D ensures an adequate supply of plasma calcium to promote calcification.
2. Vitamin C is required for normal collagen synthesis in bone matrix.
3. Vitamin A controls the differentiation to osteocalcin in bone cells, which is involved in calcium utilization from bone.
4. Vitamin K is required for the synthesis of osteocalcin in bone cells, which is involved in calcium mobilization from bone.

49–5 Concerning commonalities in the functions of the B-complex vitamins—thiamin, riboflavin, niacin, and pyridoxine:

1. These functions require the transformation of the vitamins to their respective coenzyme forms.
2. Many of the functions bring about the catabolism of the three macronutrients—carbohydrate, fat, and protein.
3. The rates of many of these functions vary with the amount of energy or protein eaten and subsequently metabolized.
4. Because of the similarity in function, the requirements of these four vitamins are very close in magnitude.

49–6 Concerning vitamin toxicity (hypervitaminosis):

1. The therapeutic use of thiamin, niacin, and riboflavin is limited by the occurrence of severe peripheral sensory neuropathy.
2. Symptoms of vitamin D toxicity include diarrhea and hypercalcemia, which may lead to calcium deposition in tissues and organs.
3. Excessive doses of vitamin E produce a hemolytic tendency, depression of liver function, and kernicterus in infants.
4. Prolonged intake of megadoses of vitamin C (2–6 g daily) is normally without serious toxicity but may cause diarrhea and renal oxalate calculi in sensitive individuals.

49–7 "Recommended intakes" of essential nutrients, including vitamins (also known as recommended dietary allowances):

1. Are based on the average physiologic requirements of normal, healthy individuals.
2. Are the amounts that will prevent a nutrient deficiency and maintain adequate tissue stores.
3. As a "safety factor" are usually set at 2 standard deviations above the average requirement.
4. Are considered sufficient for the purpose of treating specific deficiency diseases.

49–8 Which of the following vitamins are absorbed in their physiologically active form, *i.e.*, do not require additional biotransformation?

1. Vitamin K.
2. Vitamin E.
3. Vitamin C.
4. Vitamin D.

GASTROINTESTINAL SYSTEM

50–1 A clinically useful oral gastric antacid should:

1. Be of the buffering type.
2. Not be constipating.
3. Not be cathartic.
4. Preferably have systemic action.

50–2 Desirable properties of a good nonsystemic gastric antacid include:

1. The capacity to increase gastric pH to 7.4.
2. Direct inhibition of peptic enzymes.
3. Reduction of the secreted gastric acid volume.
4. Negligible absorption across the gastrointestinal mucosa.

50–3 Complications of nonsystemic antacid use include:

1. Phosphate depletion by large doses of aluminum hydroxide.
2. Constipation induced by magnesium-based antacids.
3. Reduced gastrointestinal absorption of tetracyclines in the presence of aluminum hydroxide gels.
4. Diarrhea associated with ingestion of calcium carbonate.

50–4 Effects of anticholinergic drugs (muscarinic antagonists) on functions of the gastrointestinal system include:

1. Decreased secretion of gastric acid.
2. Decreased absorption of vitamin B_{12}.
3. Reduced esophageal transit and tone.
4. Secondary histamine receptor blockade.

50–5 Histamine H_2-receptor antagonists:

1. All have an imidazole ring in common, which is important for H_2-receptor recognition.
2. Inhibit basal and stimulated gastric acid secretion.
3. Also cause H_1-receptor blockade as a side effect.
4. Secondarily decrease pepsin output and secretion.

50–6 Adverse and side effects of cimetidine include:

1. Occasional sexual dysfunction and gynecomastia in males due to antiandrogenic activity.
2. Occasional transient elevations of serum transaminases.
3. Occasional mental abnormalities mainly in patients with severe liver or renal disease or in the elderly.
4. Drug-drug interactions from inhibition of hepatic microsomal metabolism of a number of other drugs.

50–7 Omeprazole:

1. Is a substituted benzimidazole that causes powerful inhibition of gastric acid secretion.
2. Accumulates in the gastric mucosa, with a duration of action that exceeds detectable plasma levels.
3. Requires an acid environment (the parietal cell) for activation.
4. Triggers an increase in circulating gastrin in response to suppression of acid secretion.

50–8 Concerning the protection of the gastric-duodenal mucosa from acid-peptic digestion:

1. Inhibitors of E-type prostaglandins and H_2-receptor blockers have similar ulcer-healing properties.
2. Carbenoxolone increases the production of mucus and thereby helps to increase the life span of gastric mucosal cells.
3. Colloidal bismuth precipitates into a mucosa-protecting film only in the alkaline medium of the duodenum.
4. The cytoprotective action of sucrose octasulfate requires the polymerization of molecules into a viscous paste that forms a barrier by adhesion to the ulcer crater.

51–1 Concerning laxatives:

1. Most drugs in this category increase intestinal secretion of water and electrolytes and decrease their absorption.
2. The laxative action of castor oil requires prior hydrolysis of a triglyceride by pancreatic lipase to yield free ricinoleic acid.
3. Phenolphthalein must be absorbed, conjugated with glucuronide in the liver, and excreted in the bile before laxation will occur.
4. Lactulose is a nonabsorbable disaccharide that draws water into the small intestine, delivering a large fluid volume into the colon.

51–2 The chronic, habitual use of laxatives may lead to:

1. Inflammation and damage of the mucosa, known as the "cathartic colon syndrome."
2. Malabsorption of carbohydrates, fats, fat-soluble vitamins, and calcium.
3. Increased or excessive losses of proteins by the intestine.
4. Electrolyte imbalances in consequence of excessive loss of water in the stools.

51–3 Opium-containing antidiarrheal drugs:

1. Decrease gastric motility and propulsive intestinal contractions.
2. Decrease gastric and intestinal tone to the point of complete relaxation.
3. Cause more complete absorption of water from the chyme, resulting in the thickening of feces.
4. Inhibit intestinal fluid accumulation through interference with parasympathetic innervation.

51–4 The antidiarrheal drug loperamide:

1. Upon chronic use has a tendency to potentiate CNS-depressant drugs.
2. Upon chronic use produces tolerance and dependence.
3. Is less potent and slower acting than other piperidines.
4. Has a structure that is similar to diphenoxylate and haloperidol.

CHEMOTHERAPY

52–1 Concerning antimicrobial agents:

1. The mechanisms of antimicrobial action are generally based upon the concepts of "selective toxicity."
2. Most antibiotics currently used in clinical practice are semisynthetic analogs of antibiotics isolated from natural sources.
3. By definition, the term "antibiotic" is wrongly applied to substances such as sulfonamides, sulfones, and quinolones.
4. The most widely useful clinical antimicrobials, for reasons of safety and rapidity of action, are the bacteriostatic agents.

52–2 The predictably successful outcome of systemic antimicrobial chemotherapy depends on:

1. The ability of the chosen drug to be absorbed from the gastrointestinal tract.
2. The susceptibility and sensitivity of the pathogen to a chosen antimicrobial.
3. The choice of an agent with the broadest possible spectrum of antimicrobial activity.
4. The relative absence of drug effects on the host's nonpathogenic flora.

52–3 Concerning microbial resistance to antimicrobial agents:

1. Most, if not all, microorganisms are capable of developing resistance to antimicrobials.
2. R plasmid–coded resistance is inducible and transferable.
3. A typical example of induced microbial resistance is the bacterial production of penicillinase.
4. The most resistance-proof antimicrobials are the sulfonamides.

52–4 Established examples of R plasmid–coded microbial resistance to antimicrobial agents include the:

1. Prevention of transport of tetracyclines into bacterial cells.
2. Production of trimethoprim-resistant dihydrofolic acid reductase.
3. Production of sulfonamide-resistant dihydrofolic acid synthetase.
4. Enzymatic modification of aminoglycosides, reducing their affinity for bacterial ribosomes.

52–5 *In vitro* sensitivity testing:

1. Provides an important measure of antibiotic activity against one or several specific pathogens.
2. By the disc-diffusion method permits the precise calculation of required drug dosage.
3. Will indicate whether a combination of antimicrobial drugs acting together will be indifferent, antagonistic, or synergistic.
4. Is an essential diagnostic maneuver without which antimicrobial drug therapy cannot be performed.

53–1 The unique action of penicillins and cephalosporins:

1. Requires an actively growing and dividing bacterial population for maximal bactericidal activity.
2. Is an intracellular process of inhibition of amino acid transport.
3. Prevents the formation of cross-links during synthesis of bacterial cell walls.
4. Causes proteolysis of bacterial cell wall structures and the formation of spheroplasts.

53–2 Which of the following antibiotics with action on bacterial cell wall synthesis are chemically beta-lactams?

1. Penicillin G.
2. Cephalexin.
3. Imipenem.
4. Cycloserine.

53–3 The beta-lactam ring in various cell wall inhibitors:

1. Is the molecular structural portion that confers antibacterial activity.
2. Is chemically reactive, giving rise to instability of various antibiotics in acid media.
3. Is subject to hydrolysis by bacterial penicillinases, which inactivates the antibiotic.
4. Can be protected from penicillinase by combining the antibiotic with a "suicide" beta-lactamase inhibitor, such as clavulanic acid.

53–4 Which of the following penicillin preparations are acid-stable and thus well absorbed after oral administration?

1. Penicillin G.
2. Penicillin V.
3. Methicillin.
4. Ampicillin.

53–5 Which of the following penicillin preparations are sensitive to beta-lactamase and thus relatively inactive against penicillinase-producing staphylococci?

1. Penicillin G.
2. Penicillin V.
3. Ampicillin.
4. Cloxacillin.

53–6 The serum half-lives of penicillins are short because:

1. The drugs are rapidly biotransformed to inactive metabolites.
2. Interaction with bacteria causes irreversible binding to penicillin-binding proteins (PBPs).
3. Rapid redistribution into adipose tissue occurs.
4. Free drug is rapidly eliminated in the urine.

53–7 Which of the following are products of inactivation of penicillin G as a consequence of cleavage of the beta-lactam ring or thiazolidine ring?

1. Benzylpenicillenic acid.
2. Benzylpenicilloic acid.
3. Benzylpenicilloyl-protein.
4. 6-Aminopenicillanic acid.

53–8 Which of the following adverse reactions to penicillins have been observed?

1. Hypersensitivity reactions and anaphylaxis.
2. Encephalopathy associated with extremely high doses.
3. Interstitial nephritis.
4. Reversible neutropenia.

53–9 Cephalosporins differ significantly from penicillins in terms of:

1. Parent structure nucleus.
2. Ability to cause hypersensitivity reactions.
3. Exclusive reliance on parenteral administration of the newest ("third-generation") ultra-broad-spectrum drugs.
4. Distribution and elimination characteristics.

53–10 Which of the following properties prevent systemic use of bacitracin?

1. The molecule lacks a beta-lactam ring.
2. The drug is not absorbed from the gastrointestinal tract.
3. About 35% of an administered dose is biotransformed to toxic metabolites.
4. The drug's complexing with lipids causes damage to mammalian plasma membranes.

54–1 Which of the following antibiotics with action on cell membranes are classified as antifungal agents?

1. Amphotericin B.
2. Colistin.
3. Nystatin.
4. Polymyxin B.

54–2 Which are the mechanisms by which membrane-active agents cause leakage of intracellular contents and cell death?

1. Inhibition of the lipid carrier isoprenyl phosphate.
2. Reaction with phosphate groups of membrane phospholipids.
3. Binding to and cross-linking of membrane lipoproteins.
4. Interaction with membrane ergosterol and formation of channels.

54–3 Topical imidazole antifungal agents:

1. Are synthetic lipophilic compounds with low water solubility at neutral pH.
2. Inhibit cytochrome P-450 that demethylates lanosterol, the precursor of ergosterol.
3. Are the treatment of choice for fungal infections of the feet, mouth, vagina, *etc.*
4. Will cause serious hepatotoxicity when inadvertently absorbed.

54–4 Intravenous infusions of therapeutic doses of amphotericin B cause:

1. Infusion reactions due to the colloidal nature of the preparation.
2. Serious hepatic and testicular toxicity with gynecomastia.
3. Impairment of renal function through disruption of renal tubular cell membranes.
4. Induction of liver microsomal enzymes involved in the biotransformation of warfarin.

55–1 Identify the correct pairings of antibiotic and its mechanism of action on bacterial ribosome function:

1. Chloramphenicol	Inhibition of peptidyl transferase.
2. Erythromycin	Prevention of peptide chain extension.
3. Streptomycin	Misreading of the genetic code of mRNA.
4. Tetracycline	Blockade of "A"-site binding of tRNA.

55–2 Concerning the kinetics of aminoglycosides:

1. Absorption from the gastrointestinal tract is minimal, but rapid after intramuscular administration.
2. The drugs are all highly protein-bound (in excess of 70%).
3. Excretion is primarily by renal glomerular filtration.
4. The serum elimination half-life ranges from 6 to 10 hours.

55–3 Important dose-limiting adverse reactions to aminoglycosides are:

1. Vestibular toxicity of streptomycin.
2. Cochlear toxicity of neomycin.
3. Nephrotoxicity of tobramycin.
4. Anaphylactic reactions with gentamicin.

55–4 Tetracyclines:

1. Are acid-stable, which provides for rapid and complete gastrointestinal absorption.
2. Are poorly absorbed in the presence of milk, milk products, and some cations (calcium, magnesium, iron) in the gastrointestinal tract.
3. Have half-lives in the 1–2 hour range.
4. Are eliminated mostly by renal glomerular filtration and variable degrees of biliary excretion.

55–5 Adverse reactions to tetracyclines include:

1. Gastrointestinal disturbances (nausea, vomiting, diarrhea).
2. Photosensitivity (exaggerated sunburn reactions).
3. Discoloration of children's tooth enamel (deposition in teeth and bones).
4. Tooth and bone abnormalities in the offspring of mothers treated with tetracyclines during pregnancy.

55–6 Chloramphenicol:

1. Is bactericidal against most microorganisms.
2. Cannot be administered by mouth because of its extremely bad taste.
3. Is excreted to the largest extent in unchanged active form by glomerular filtration.
4. Must in part be conjugated with glucuronic acid for tubular secretion.

55–7 Concerning adverse reactions to chloramphenicol:

1. An infrequent but most feared complication of therapy is aplastic anemia.
2. Dose-dependent bone marrow toxicity may cause reversible depression of the hematopoietic system.
3. Immaturity of the hepatic glucuronyl transferase system is the cause of the neonatal gray baby syndrome.
4. Hypersensitivity reactions of the anaphylactoid type are frequently observed.

55–8 Erythromycin and clindamycin:

1. Are useful alternative antibiotics to treat staphylococcal and streptococcal infections in penicillin-allergic patients.
2. Are both destroyed by acid hydrolysis in the stomach, which requires special oral formulations.
3. Cause gastrointestinal disturbances as the most prominent side effects.
4. Are rapidly excreted unchanged by renal mechanisms, only a small portion being biotransformed.

55–9 Which of the following antibiotics belong to the group of aminoglycosides?

1. Amikacin.
2. Lincomycin.
3. Netilmicin.
4. Spectinomycin.

55–10 The tetracyclines are all derivatives of:

1. Aminoglycoside.
2. Fluoroquinolone.
3. Isonicotinic acid hydrazide.
4. Naphthacenecarboxamide.

56–1 The antifungal agent griseofulvin:

1. Inhibits fungal DNA production, but it is also active against mammalian cells by inhibiting mitosis.
2. Is distributed preferentially to keratinized tissues, where it exerts topical effects after systemic administration.
3. May induce liver microsomal enzymes and thus increase the biotransformation of warfarin.
4. Is itself subject to enhanced inactivation through enzyme induction by barbiturates.

56–2 Concerning flucytosine (5-fluorocytosine):

1. The drug requires *in vivo* deamination to 5-fluorouracil before it can inhibit nucleic acid replication in susceptible yeast cells.
2. Approximately 90% of absorbed flucytosine is excreted in the urine as the active 5-fluorouracil.
3. Flucytosine is most useful in the systemic treatment of severe cutaneous and mucocutaneous candidiasis.
4. Adverse reactions are very infrequent because of the drug's high specificity for fungal organisms.

56–3 Concerning the treatment of tuberculosis:

1. Only drugs that are direct inhibitors of nucleic acid biosynthesis can be expected to act against *Mycobacterium tuberculosis.*
2. Effective therapy usually employs the concomitant or sequential use of two or more drugs in order to delay the emergence of microbial resistance.
3. The drugs in common use are all synthetic compounds specifically designed for targeted distribution into foci of infection.
4. Treatment is often complicated by the appearance of toxicity that can limit the required duration of therapy and the effective doses of antitubercular drugs.

56–4 Isoniazid (INH):

1. Is inactivated mainly by N-acetyltransferase to acetylisoniazid, followed by hydrolysis to isonicotinic acid and acetylhydrazine.
2. Acetylation is under genetic control, with rapid and slow acetylators distributed fairly evenly in the world's human population.
3. Toxicity consists of neurotoxic and hepatotoxic manifestations, the latter being more prevalent in older patients.
4. Is used only after other less toxic drugs have failed because its complicated biotransformation requirements and toxicity are distinct disadvantages.

56–5 Rifampin and ethambutol:

1. Are both antituberculous macrocyclic antibiotics.
2. Are seldom used alone, but in combination with other antituberculous agents.
3. Have a common spectrum of toxicity characterized by visual disturbances.
4. Have uses in infections caused by atypical mycobacteria and unrelated pathogens.

56–6 The fluoroquinolones norfloxacin and ciprofloxacin:

1. Inhibit microbial DNA gyrase.
2. Are considered bactericidal against susceptible microorganisms.
3. Have favorable half-lives for convenient twice-a-day administration.
4. Are eliminated unchanged in the urine.

56–7 Concerning the class of antifol antibacterial agents:

1. These drugs are all synthetic compounds with well-defined mechanisms of selective antibacterial toxicity.
2. Their common mechanism of action is inhibition of bacterial dihydrofolic acid reductase.
3. In historic terms the group of sulfanilamide derivatives were the first antibacterials that could be administered systemically.
4. The gastrointestinal absorption of antifols is generally compromised by ready acid hydrolysis in the stomach.

56–8 Concerning currently used sulfonamides:

1. Preferred usage is in fixed-dose combination with trimethoprim.
2. Hypersensitivity reactions and hematologic toxicity may occur.
3. The main elimination mechanism is acetylation to inactive conjugates, excreted by the kidneys.
4. Renal damage from crystallization is frequent because of poor water solubility of the drugs.

56–9 The antibacterial chemotherapeutic value of trimethoprim rests upon the fact that:

1. Para-aminobenzoic acid is required for the synthesis of bacterial cell walls.
2. The drug is inactivated rapidly in the human liver, but not by bacteria.
3. It is a competitive antagonist of folic acid.
4. It has a much higher affinity for bacterial than for mammalian dihydrofolic acid reductase.

56–10 Sulfones:

1. Have considerable human toxicity because of irreversible binding to dihydrofolic acid reductase.
2. Are the primary drugs used in the treatment of leprosy and some forms of chloroquine-resistant malaria.
3. Must be administered together with high doses of folinic acid to lessen toxicity.
4. Undergo a variety of phase 2 biotransformation reactions, some of which are required for urinary excretion.

57–1 Malaria patients with a genetic deficiency of glucose-6-phosphate dehydrogenase (G-6-PD) may have hemolytic drug reactions with the use of:

1. Chlorguanide.
2. Pyrimethamine.
3. Tetracycline.
4. Primaquine.

57–2 Concerning drugs used in the prophylaxis and treatment of malaria:

1. Quinine, chloroquine, and the sulfonamides are classified as blood schizonticides.
2. The drug of choice for the treatment of malaria, except where resistant strains occur, is chloroquine.
3. Primaquine acts on the hepatic phase of a malaria parasite's development.
4. When taken exactly as directed, blood schizonticides will confer absolute protection against malaria infection.

57–3 Which of the following are relatively common side effects from large doses of antimalarials?

1. Chloroquine: dizziness, reversible vision disturbances.
2. Mefloquine: gastrointestinal upset.
3. Pyrimethamine: possible teratogenic effects.
4. Quinidine: tinnitus, headache.

57–4 Metronidazole:

1. Is used to treat amebiasis, giardiasis, and trichomoniasis.
2. In high and prolonged dosage is carcinogenic in mice.
3. Causes gastrointestinal upset as a common adverse effect.
4. Has been associated with disulfiram-like reactions.

57–5 Which of the following drugs are used in the treatment of *Enterobius vermicularis* (pinworm)?

1. Mebendazole.
2. Thiabendazole.
3. Pyrantel pamoate.
4. Niclosamide.

57–6 Concerning mechanisms of action of antiparasitic drugs:

1. Mebendazole inhibits DNA synthesis in parasites.
2. Pyrantel pamoate causes spastic paralysis of intestinal worms.
3. Piperazine citrate increases the permeability of worm cell membranes to calcium ions.
4. Pyrvinium pamoate inhibits glucose uptake by susceptible parasites.

57–7 Concerning commonly observed adverse effects of antiparasitic drugs:

1. Pyrvinium pamoate colors the stool orange, staining underwear and bed sheets.
2. Thiabendazole produces gastrointestinal upset, dizziness, and headache.
3. Piperazine citrate lowers the seizure threshold; it is contraindicated in patients with seizure disorders.
4. Diloxanide furoate produces subacute myelo-optic neuropathy (SMON) after prolonged use.

58–1 Concerning mechanisms of action of antiviral drugs:

1. Amantadine interferes with viral uncoating.
2. Adenine arabinoside (Ara-A, vidarabine) competitively inhibits viral DNA polymerase.
3. Ribavirin blocks capping of viral mRNA.
4. Zidovudine (AZT) acts as a chain terminator of DNA synthesis.

58–2 Amantadine:

1. Is effective in the prophylaxis and treatment of type A influenza.
2. Undergoes extensive biotransformation to active metabolites.
3. Is used in the treatment of Parkinson's disease.
4. Causes bone marrow depression and liver toxicity.

58–3 Accepted clinical indications for the use of idoxuridine (IDU) are:

1. Herpes encephalitis (systemic use).
2. Herpes genitalis (topical use).
3. Respiratory syncytial virus (aerosol).
4. Herpetic keratitis (topical use).

58–4 Vidarabine (Ara-A):

1. Is the drug of choice to treat cytomegalovirus infections in compromised hosts.
2. Is poorly water soluble and therefore must be administered in large volumes.
3. Is only minimally biotransformed; therefore it is excreted largely unchanged in the urine.
4. May cause CNS side effects such as tremor, ataxia, paresthesias, and confusion.

58–5 Accepted clinical indications for the use of acyclovir are:

1. Herpes genitalis infections (topical use).
2. Genital herpes simplex infections (oral use).
3. Varicella-zoster infections (intravenous use).
4. Cytomegalovirus infections in transplant patients (intramuscular use).

58–6 Zidovudine (AZT):

1. Is a guanine derivative that was first introduced in 1960 as an antineoplastic drug.
2. Significantly decreases the frequency of opportunistic infections and the mortality in patients with human immunodeficiency virus (HIV) infection.
3. Is poorly absorbed from the gastrointestinal tract because of its instability at low gastric pH.
4. Causes anemia, leukopenia, neutropenia, and decreased vitamin B_{12} levels in the majority of treated patients.

58–7 Interferons cause a range of biologic and biochemical effects, some of which are utilized in the prevention and treatment of disease, such as:

1. Antiviral action.
2. Antineoplastic action.
3. Immunosuppressant action.
4. Antibacterial action.

59–1 Concerning the defining terminology of infection control:

1. Antisepsis: destruction of bacteria, or limitation of their growth, by application of chemicals to living tissues.
2. Disinfection: destruction of bacteria (except spore forms) by application of agents or processes to inanimate objects.
3. Sterilization: destruction of all microorganisms (including spore forms) by physical or chemical processes.
4. Sanitation: reduction to safe levels (that meet public health requirements) of the number of bacterial contaminants in a given environment.

59–2 Ethyl and isopropyl alcohol kill vegetative bacteria most effectively:

1. When colored with methylene blue.
2. When 0.1% sodium nitrate is added.
3. At 95% concentration.
4. At 60–70% concentrations.

59–3 Concerning iodine preparations:

1. Iodine compounds have broad activity against bacteria, spore forms, yeasts, and viruses.
2. When combined with surfactants, iodine is solubilized as micellar aggregates.
3. Iodophors are less painful, staining, irritating, and allergenic than tincture of iodine.
4. When used as a skin antiseptic, povidone-iodine will effectively kill resident and transient flora for at least 24 hours.

59–4 Concerning phenol derivatives:

1. Carbolic acid was used by Lister to introduce the concept of aseptic surgery in the mid-19th century.
2. All preparations in use today are substitutions with greatly increased bactericidal activity and reduced toxicity.
3. Hexachlorophene is employed to good advantage as a preoperative antiseptic bath or shower and as a presurgical scrub.
4. Modern phenol derivatives are safe to use in the pediatric setting because of their negligible systemic toxicity.

59–5 Concerning heavy metal derivatives:

1. The main microbial cellular targets for silver salts are thiol groups and enzymes with thiol groups.
2. The topical use of 1% silver nitrate to prevent neonatal gonococcal conjunctivitis is an outmoded, inadequate, and toxic procedure.
3. Silver sulfadiazine utilizes the combined antibacterial spectra of silver ions and sulfonamides in the antisepsis of burn patients.
4. Although only bacteriostatic, mercurochrome has remained a skin antiseptic of proven value.

60–1 Considering the nature of neoplastic disease and the mechanisms of cytotoxic action, which of the following dose schedules of antineoplastic drug therapy would be expected to achieve maximum tumor cell kill?

1. Low-dose continuous.
2. High-dose continuous.
3. Alternating high and low doses.
4. High-dose intermittent.

60–2 Concerning the principal mechanisms of antineoplastic drug action:

1. Mitotic inhibitors inhibit spindle formation (*i.e.*, cause metaphase arrest) in cells undergoing mitosis.
2. Antimetabolites inhibit nucleic acid formation for DNA synthesis.
3. Alkylating agents cause cross-linking of DNA with subsequent inhibition of strand separation.
4. Antibiotics cause misreading of the genetic code of mRNA.

60–3 Which of the following antineoplastic drugs are classified as antimetabolites?

1. Cytosine arabinoside (Ara-C).
2. 5-Fluorouracil (5-FU).
3. 6-Mercaptopurine (6-MP).
4. Methotrexate.

60–4 All alkylating agents:

1. Are highly reactive substances that combine with pyrimidine and purine bases in DNA.
2. Are strictly cycle-dependent, acting on cells only during cell division.
3. Produce bone marrow depression as the principal dose-limiting toxicity.
4. Must undergo *in vivo* hepatic biotransformation to alkylating metabolites.

60–5 In addition to myelosuppression and neutropenia, alkylating agents have other common toxicities, such as:

1. Peripheral neuropathy.
2. Nausea and vomiting.
3. Hepatitis.
4. Alopecia of varying degrees.

60–6 The lethal toxicity associated with very high doses of methotrexate can be avoided with administrations of folinic acid because:

1. Folinic acid inhibits methotrexate absorption.
2. Methotrexate binds competitively to folinic acid.
3. The activity of dihydrofolic acid reductase is stimulated by folinic acid.
4. Folinic acid does not require dihydrofolic acid reductase for activity.

60–7 Tamoxifen:

1. Is a nonsteroidal antiandrogen.
2. Induces DNA and RNA synthesis.
3. Is very useful in the treatment of breast cancer.
4. Therapy requires mineralocorticoid supplementation.

60–8 When comparing the two vinca alkaloids, vincristine and vinblastine:

1. The half-life of vinblastine is about 10 times longer than that of vincristine.
2. The predominant dose-limiting toxicity is neuropathy for vincristine and myelosuppression for vinblastine.
3. Vincristine can cause a syndrome of inappropriate ADH secretion (SIADH).
4. Vincristine is preferentially given orally, whereas vinblastine can on occasion also be injected.

60–9 Significant limiting factors of antineoplastic chemotherapy include:

1. The very complicated unconventional routes required for effective drug administration.
2. The low therapeutic index of antineoplastic drugs.
3. The inability of most drugs to distribute to tumor sites in effective cytotoxic concentrations.
4. The high probability of tumor cells developing resistance.

61–1 The objective of immunosuppressive chemotherapy in organ transplantation is to:

1. Destroy the surge of immune cell proliferation at the time of transplantation.
2. Allow immune rebound between monthly high-dose suppressant drug therapy.
3. Maintain long-term immune cell destruction with low daily doses of suppressant drugs.
4. Cause permanent atrophy of lymphoid tissues with high doses of cytotoxic drugs.

61–2 Major immunosuppressant properties of glucocorticosteroids (*e.g.*, prednisone) are:

1. Reduction of size and lymphoid content of lymph nodes and spleen.
2. Suppression of inflammatory responses and cell-mediated immunity.
3. Destruction (*i.e.*, lysis) of certain T-cell subsets.
4. Decrease of specific antibody concentrations and antibody responses.

61–3 Azathioprine:

1. Is an analog of the antineoplastic drug methotrexate.
2. Is used for immunosuppression in relation to organ transplantation.
3. Activates natural killer (cytotoxic) cells.
4. Toxicity is primarily myelosuppression.

61–4 The fungal antibiotic cyclosporine A:

1. Interferes with immune response regulation by inhibiting the production of interleukin-2.
2. Affects cell-mediated cytolysis in graft-host reactions.
3. Is effective in suppressing delayed-type hypersensitivity.
4. Has major dose-limiting toxicity on bone marrow function.

SPECIAL TOPICS

62–1 Impairment of hepatic circulation may decrease the delivery of drugs to liver cells and also decrease the supply of oxygen for hepatic biotransformation processes. The rate of elimination from the body of which of the following drugs would likely decrease as a consequence?

1. Digoxin (cardiac glycoside).
2. Digitoxin (cardiac glycoside).
3. Isoflurane (inhalational general anesthetic).
4. Halothane (inhalational general anesthetic).

62–2 Decreased plasma protein concentrations as a result of chronic liver disease can raise the free fraction of normally extensively protein-bound drugs, which in turn can increase their hepatic uptake. Which of the following drugs were shown to be affected in this way?

1. Diazepam.
2. Phenytoin.
3. Propranolol.
4. Tolbutamide.

62–3 Severe liver disease (*e.g.*, active cirrhosis) may cause reductions in hepatic content and activity of cytochrome P-450, N- and O-demethylases, pseudocholinesterase, and glucose-6-phosphate dehydrogenase. The resulting deficits in biotransformation, demanding dosage reductions, would affect:

1. Meperidine.
2. Phenylbutazone.
3. Propranolol.
4. Penicillin G.

62–4 Biliary obstruction may significantly increase the duration of action of drugs that depend on biliary secretion for much of their elimination, such as:

1. Acetaminophen.
2. Digitoxin.
3. Ibuprofen.
4. Thiopental.

62–5 Direct hepatotoxic damage (liver cell necrosis) may be caused by:

1. Acetaminophen in excess of glutathione conjugating capacity, producing a highly reactive metabolite.
2. Halothane *via* hypoxia-induced cytochrome P-450 reduction to a membrane-bound free radical.
3. α-Methyldopa *via* the formation of an epoxide intermediary metabolite acting as an arylating agent.
4. Tetracyclines through interference with cell protein synthesis and subsequent inhibition of triglyceride transport.

62–6 Alcohol-induced fatty liver:

1. Results mainly from a metabolic increase in hepatic NADH, which stimulates the synthesis of fatty acids and accumulation of neutral fat in the liver.
2. Leads directly to hepatic fibrosis and cirrhosis.
3. Is usually accompanied by elevations of serum lactate and glycerol-3-phosphate.
4. Is the single most important predisposing risk factor in the "excess mortality" of alcoholics.

62–7 Widely accepted causes of alcoholic hepatocellular necrosis are:

1. Selective precipitation of cellular proteins.
2. Focal hypoxia from excessively low oxygen tensions in centrilobular areas.
3. Abnormally depressed or absent thyroid hormone function.
4. Acetaldehyde-mediated immunologic events at cell surfaces.

62–8 Contributing factors in the development of alcoholic cirrhosis of the liver (hepatic fibrosis) after prolonged alcohol abuse may be:

1. Stimulation of fibrogenesis and collagen synthesis by alcohol itself.
2. Repeated episodes of liver cell necrosis in the centrilobular areas.
3. Portal hypertension that induces collagen accumulation in Disse's space.
4. Chronic vitamin B complex deficiency, protein deficiency, and recurrent bouts of hypoglycemia.

63–1 Which of the following drugs were reported to be carcinogenic in human target organs?

1. Acetophenetidin (phenacetin) in the kidney.
2. Chloramphenicol in the hematopoietic system.
3. Phenytoin in the lymphoreticular system.
4. Diethylstilbestrol in the vagina.

63–2 Metabolic activation of precarcinogens into ultimate carcinogens:

1. Is a process of biotransforming unreactive substances into chemically reactive (electron-deficient) products.
2. Is carried out primarily by microbial flora within the mammalian host.
3. Usually involves more than one enzymatic step.
4. Is a "model" of chemically induced tumor formation in rodents that does not occur in humans.

63–3 Concerning initiation of neoplastic transformation:

1. Covalent binding of an ultimate carcinogen to DNA can alter the genetic message.
2. A genetic lesion may be "fixed," to be inherited by all progeny of the altered cell.
3. The key event is believed to be the conversion of a normal proto-oncogene by a carcinogen into an oncogene.
4. All chemically induced mutations will eventually lead to cancer after varying periods of latency.

63–4 The detection of carcinogenicity:

1. Is relatively easy because of well-established cause-effect relationships.
2. Is greatly facilitated by large-scale testing and screening of suspect chemicals for mutagenic properties.
3. Makes exclusive use of highly specialized *in vitro* systems that provide more specific results than was possible *in vivo*.
4. Rests on carefully designed human epidemiologic studies for ultimate "proof."

63–5 Concerning dose-response considerations in carcinogenesis:

1. Responses at all carcinogen dose levels have been adequately defined in rodents for extrapolation to a human population.
2. A "safe" dose for carcinogens can be calculated with certainty from animal dose-response curves.
3. Mathematical models have been constructed with which the specific carcinogenic mechanism of each agent can be determined for risk assessment.
4. Regulatory decisions about many potential carcinogens must be made without conclusive experimental evidence of risk.

64–1 Concerning the assessment of human teratologic risk:

1. Most teratologic studies are restricted to the perinatal period without evaluation of maturational processes.
2. Teratologic evaluation often depends upon retrospective epidemiologic studies.
3. Fetal toxicity of most drugs can be assessed only after their use in the general population.
4. Teratologic risks can be reduced to some extent by preclinical animal studies and *in vitro* tests.

64–2 Concerning critical periods of susceptibility to teratogenic agents during human prenatal development:

1. The critical period that is most susceptible to the production of anomalies is the time from fertilization to blastocyst implantation.
2. Central nervous system development is highly susceptible during the first 3 weeks of the embryonic period and remains sensitive until the time of birth.
3. The early weeks of organogenesis were shown to be the most sensitive to functional teratogenesis.
4. The development of heart, limbs, and palate ceases to be susceptible to teratogenic agents after the first trimester of pregnancy.

64–3 Concerning teratogenic specificity:

1. Teratogens will cause markedly different anomalies depending on the phase of fetal development.
2. The most "specific" teratogens, causing a limited number of anomalies, are the cytotoxic anticancer drugs.
3. Teratogenic dose specificity can affect both the type and frequency of anomalies.
4. Most agents that are teratogenic in the last trimester of pregnancy are carcinogenic in postnatal life.

64–4 Concerning chemical mechanisms of teratogenesis:

1. Fetal toxicity of a drug can be due to an exaggeration of the (reversible) pharmacologic activity for which the drug is used therapeutically.
2. Fetal toxicity of a drug can be caused by the (generally irreversible) action of a reactive intermediate, unrelated to the pharmacologic mechanism and therapeutic effect.
3. Environmental chemicals may have fetal toxicity by reversibly binding to a receptor or by irreversible interaction of a reactive intermediate with fetal tissues.
4. In order to be able to react with fetal tissues, a drug radical must first inhibit the fetal cyclooxygenase pathway of eicosanoid synthesis.

64–5 Among the *in vitro* tests for screening teratogenic chemicals are:

1. Cells in culture as a rapid indicator of chemical teratogenicity.
2. Embryonic organs in culture as a measure of developmental processes.
3. Whole embryos in culture for mechanistic studies of chemical teratogenicity.
4. "Artificial embryos" for the quick and inexpensive detection of teratogenic potential for large numbers of chemicals.

65–1 Identify the correct definitions of allergic or hypersensitivity drug reactions:

1. Type 1 = immediate or anaphylactic; interaction of allergen (drug) with IgE antibody; release of chemical mediators.
2. Type 2 = complement fixation (cytotoxic); hapten (drug) and blood cell surface protein constituting complete antigen, causing formation of specific antibody; subsequent antigen-antibody reactions with complement fixation leading to blood cell lysis.
3. Type 3 = immune-complex-mediated (cytotoxic); deposition of antigen-antibody complexes on tissue cells; complement activation causes release of lysosomal enzymes and tissue destruction.
4. Type 4 = cell-mediated; direct interaction between allergen (drug) and sensitized lymphocytes; release of lymphokines.

65–2 Dose-related adverse drug reactions:

1. Are the most commonly encountered drug reactions.
2. Show direct proportionality to the administered dose; they respond to dosage adjustments.
3. May have indirect or contributing causes when drug elimination is impaired.
4. Can usually not be predicted from animal toxicologic studies.

65–3 Adverse drug reactions unrelated to dose:

1. Are frequently associated with liver and/or kidney dysfunction.
2. Are usually due to an increased susceptibility of the patient.
3. Have very low mortality because of the certainty with which they can be predicted.
4. Comprise most of the drug reactions with a pharmacogenetic basis.

65–4 Concerning some factors associated with adverse drug reactions, as suggested by epidemiologic studies:

1. Older subjects (> 60 years of age) are more susceptible to adverse drug reactions than younger ones.
2. Gender differences are statistically not significant when psychological factors are excluded.
3. Patients on multiple-drug therapy have an increased probability of developing adverse drug reactions.
4. Careful drug monitoring studies indicated that the patient's disease state has no contributing influence on adverse drug reactions.

65–5 An adverse event is deemed to be definitely associated with the administration of a particular drug, if the reaction:

1. Follows a reasonable temporal sequence after drug administration, or after drug levels in the body have been established.
2. Follows a known response pattern.
3. Is confirmed by improvement on removal of the drug and by reappearance on rechallenge.
4. Cannot be explained by the known characteristics of the patient's disease.

66–1 In animals, drug-induced decreases in serotonergic activity will cause behavioral changes such as:

1. Increased sensitivity to painful stimuli.
2. Much delayed acquisition of avoidance responses.
3. Increased aggressive behavior.
4. Abolition of sex-related behaviors.

66–2 In animals, modification of central catecholamine or cholinergic function by drugs produces these characteristic behavioral effects:

1. Administration of reserpine leads to profoundly decreased spontaneous locomotor activity.
2. Reduction of catecholamine levels with 6-hydroxydopamine increases aggressiveness and fighting, which can be antagonized by apomorphine.
3. Physostigmine causes an animal to appear to be sleeping while the EEG is that of an awake animal.
4. Application of norepinephrine [noradrenaline] to certain hypothalamic areas causes profound aversion to food to the point of starvation.

66–3 In animals:

1. Low doses of strychnine and strychnine-like drugs inhibit the normal acquisition of visual and maze-learning tasks.
2. Injections of amphetamine improve learning, perhaps through effects on attention mechanisms.
3. Vasopressin causes rapid extinction of learned shock-avoidance responses.
4. Anticholinergics impair learning; increased cholinergic activity appears to facilitate it.

66–4 Concerning the reinforcing properties of drugs in animal models:

1. Pentobarbital and diazepam act as negative reinforcers by inhibiting drug-taking behavior.
2. Chlorpromazine, amitriptyline, and nalorphine strengthen drug-taking behavior.
3. LSD and tetrahydrocannabinol are positive reinforcers that generate avid self-administration.
4. Studies of drug self-administration in experimental animals, although important, have certain limitations in the assessment of human drug abuse potential.

67–1 The W.H.O. Expert Committee in 1964 defined "drug addiction" as:

1. An overpowering desire or need to continue taking a drug and to obtain it by any means.
2. A tendency to increase the dose of the drug.
3. A psychological and sometimes physical dependence on the drug's effects.
4. A state of chronic intoxication from which the patient cannot be withdrawn.

67–2 Concerning various forms of tolerance:

1. Metabolic tolerance implies the increasing production of active metabolites.
2. Target tissue tolerance arises from adaptive tissue changes that tend to offset the drug effects.
3. Target tissue tolerance is always accompanied by pathologic changes in the respective tissues.
4. Metabolic cross-tolerance is important for drugs that are biotransformed by hepatic microsomal enzymes.

67–3 Physical dependence:

1. Is demonstrated by the abolition of a withdrawal reaction with a fresh dose of the drug.
2. Will not occur if the drug does not cause a morphine type of withdrawal reaction.
3. Can be transferred between drugs within a cross-tolerant group (*i.e.*, cross-dependence).
4. On the same drug cannot be reacquired after the drug has been stopped and normal sensitivity has been restored.

67–4 Concerning the use of pharmacologic agents in the treatment of drug dependence:

1. The goal of treatment is to stop the undesired drug-taking response from being self-reinforcing.
2. In methadone maintenance of heroin addicts a less reinforcing drug is substituted for a strongly reinforcing one.
3. Specific blockers can prevent the usual reinforcing drug effects and thus may lead to extinction of the conditioned behavior.
4. Aversive agents may interact with the drug to produce unpleasant instead of rewarding effects.

67–5 Identify the appropriate pharmacologic agents contained in the following psychoactive substances:

1. Betel—arecoline (nicotine-like).
2. Kaapi—indole derivatives (hallucinogens).
3. Khat—cathinone (central stimulant).
4. Mescal—opioids (morphine-like).

68–1 Concerning placental drug transfer:

1. The placental barrier is impermeable to drugs with molecular weights greater than 1000.
2. The transfer of inhalational anesthetics at delivery is generally determined by placental blood flow, reaching maternal-fetal equilibrium within minutes.
3. At fetal blood pH, basic compounds tend to be trapped on the fetal side of the placenta.
4. The fetus at delivery has lower total serum proteins than the mother, which leads to decreased albumin binding of salicylate.

68–2 Which of the following functions are usually not fully developed at birth, with possible consequences for drug clearance?

1. Hepatic cytochrome P-450–dependent monooxygenation.
2. Hepatic conjugation with glucuronide.
3. Cholinergic receptor function in ileum and heart.
4. Renal glomerular filtration rate and renal plasma flow.

68–3 The incidence of respiratory distress syndrome (RDS) in premature infants will be reduced by prenatal (prophylactic) administration to the mother of:

1. Digoxin.
2. Cromolyn sodium [sodium cromoglycate].
3. Theophylline.
4. Betamethasone.

68–4 Concerning the use of theophylline in the management of neonatal apnea:

1. Respiration appears to be stimulated by augmentation of CO_2 responsiveness and improved diaphragmatic contractility.
2. The half-life of theophylline in the newborn is short because of efficient N-demethylation.
3. Conversion to caffeine occurs via active methylation, with accumulation of caffeine to levels approaching those of theophylline.
4. The half-life of the metabolite caffeine in the newborn is approximately 10 hours.

68–5 Prostaglandins from fetal tissues and placenta:

1. May cause alterations in uterine and placental blood flow.
2. Influence organ differentiation, especially when produced locally.
3. Mediate fetal and placental hormone production and release.
4. Are responsible for persistent ductus arteriosus in infants of low birth weight.

69–1 Significant average changes in body function (males and females) from age 20 to age 80 were demonstrated for:

1. Vital capacity −60%.
2. Glomerular filtration rate −50%.
3. Cardiac output −30%.
4. Conduction velocity +20%.

69–2 Significant average changes in body fluid composition (males and females) from age 20 to age 80 were demonstrated for:

1. Plasma volume +10%.
2. Total body water +15%.
3. Extracellular fluid +20%.
4. Plasma albumin −10%.

69–3 Possibly important pharmacokinetic changes in the elderly include:

1. Decreased output of gastric acid, affecting ionization and solubility of some drugs.
2. Increased fraction of total body weight consisting of adipose tissue, possibly affecting distribution of some drugs.
3. Multifactorial decrease in hepatic clearance of some drugs.
4. Reduced glomerular filtration rate and renal blood flow, possibly prolonging the elimination half-life of some drugs.

69–4 Possibly important pharmacodynamic changes in the elderly include:

1. Multifactorial increase in digitalis sensitivity.
2. Reduced incidence of side effects of analgesics.
3. Increased sensitivity to anticoagulants such as warfarin.
4. Decreased response to CNS-active drugs, with generally fewer side effects.

69–5 Strong association of increasing patient age to frequency of adverse drug reactions has been demonstrated for:

1. Diazepam.
2. Lidocaine.
3. Heparin.
4. Propranolol.

70–1 Concerning patient compliance with prescribed treatment schedules:

1. The compliance rate for short-term preventive medication is usually twice as good as for long-term preventive medication.
2. The larger the number of different drugs to be taken, the poorer the compliance.
3. The patient's perception of the disease and the efficacy of appropriate drug therapy tend to improve compliance.
4. Medications with unpleasant side effects or inconvenient treatment schedules generally decrease compliance.

70–2 Pharmacokinetic sources of variation in drug response include:

1. Genetically determined alterations in biotransformation.
2. Genetically determined abnormal tissue responses to drugs.
3. The presence of inflammatory conditions that alter the permeability of drug barriers.
4. Coexisting disease processes that alter the number or distribution of specific drug receptors.

70–3 Concerning drug dosage in children of different ages:

1. The required dose for a given individual is strictly proportional to the body weight, as shown by the universal use of "mg/kg."
2. A 12-year-old boy, by rule of thumb, will likely require one half of an adult dose.
3. The calculation of an infant's dose on the basis of age (Young's rule) assumes 60 kg adult weight and 6 kg infant weight, *i.e.*, 10%.
4. The calculation of children's doses by body surface area approximates metabolically active mass and corresponding surface area relative to a 65-kg adult.

71–1 The toxicity rating "very toxic" in terms of poisoning potential (LD_{50} = 50–500 mg/kg) applies to:

1. Methanol.
2. Acetylsalicylic acid (aspirin).
3. Digoxin.
4. Phenobarbital.

71–2 The toxicity rating "super toxic" in terms of poisoning potential (LD_{50} < 5 mg/kg) applies to:

1. Potassium cyanide.
2. Nicotine.
3. d-Tubocurarine.
4. Malathion.

71–3 Concerning modifiers of manifestations of toxicity:

1. *Age:* young children show more severe signs of toxicity than adults when poisoned with antihistamines, ethanol, salicylates.
2. *Exposure duration:* acute exposure to benzene results in CNS depression; chronic exposure is associated with hematologic changes.
3. *Metabolic activation:* requiring activation to cause toxicity are acetaminophen, methanol, and organophosphates.
4. *Nutrition:* the presence of food in the stomach consistently enhances the absorption (*i.e.,* toxicity) of orally administered compounds.

72–1 Concerning possible measures to decrease the gastrointestinal absorption of ingested toxins:

1. The drug of choice to induce emesis (vomiting) in the majority of subjects is orally administered syrup of ipecac.
2. The safest and most effective method for the removal of solid toxic substances from the stomach is gastric lavage.
3. Orally administered activated charcoal mixed with water binds toxins within the gastrointestinal tract and reduces their absorption.
4. Ingested strong alkalis and acids are effectively neutralized with weak acids and alkalis, respectively, for harmless excretion.

72–2 Concerning antidotal therapy:

1. Morphine-induced sedation, respiratory depression, and miosis are antagonized by naloxone, which competes reversibly with μ and κ opioid receptors in brain and spinal cord.
2. The effects of carbamate insecticide poisoning are antagonized by atropine, which lessens the toxic symptoms manifested as "cholinergic syndrome."
3. Administration of sodium nitrite in acute cyanide poisoning creates large circulating pools of ferric iron that cause removal of cyanide ion from the toxic cytox-FeCN complex.
4. Intoxication with ethylene glycol (an antifreeze) is treated with ethanol, which prevents metabolic conversion of ethylene glycol to its more toxic metabolites.

72–3 Which of the following are recognized agents for the treatment by chelation of metal intoxications?

1. Dimercaprol (BAL) for the treatment of arsenic poisoning.
2. Calcium disodium EDTA ($CaNa_2EDTA$) for the treatment of lead poisoning.
3. Deferoxamine for the treatment of iron poisoning.
4. Penicillamine for the treatment of cadmium poisoning.

72–4 As a treatment of overdose, the renal excretion of which of the following drugs can be increased by alkalinization of the urine ("ionized diuresis")?

1. Amphetamines.
2. Phenobarbital.
3. Quinidine.
4. Salicylates.

72–5 Which of the following toxins can be absorbed through the unbroken skin?

1. Carbon tetrachloride.
2. Nicotine.
3. Phenol.
4. Tetraethyl lead.

SECTION III

ANSWERS

Except for questions 6–9 and 6–10 (pharmacokinetic exercises), these answers are all based on the common answer key printed at the top of each questions page. The numbering conforms to the compound numbering (by chapter) used throughout Section II.

1–1 = B
1–2 = D
1–3 = A
1–4 = B
1–5 = D
1–6 = D

2–1 = E
2–2 = D
2–3 = E
2–4 = E
2–5 = D
2–6 = E
2–7 = E
2–8 = A
2–9 = C
2–10 = A
2–11 = E
2–12 = C

3–1 = E
3–2 = D
3–3 = A
3–4 = A
3–5 = C
3–6 = A
3–7 = A
3–8 = B
3–9 = B
3–10 = A

4–1 = A
4–2 = D
4–3 = E
4–4 = C
4–5 = A
4–6 = B
4–7 = E
4–8 = E
4–9 = B
4–10 = E

5–1 = B
5–2 = B
5–3 = A
5–4 = C
5–5 = E
5–6 = B
5–7 = C
5–8 = A

6–1 = B
6–2 = A
6–3 = E
6–4 = A
6–5 = A
6–6 = B
6–7 = C
6–8 = A
6–9a = 2
6–9b = 3
6–9c = 4
6–9d = 3
6–9e = 2
6–9f = 3
6–10a = 1
6–10b = 4
6–10c = 3
6–10d = 4

7–1 = E
7–2 = A
7–3 = A
7–4 = C
7–5 = E
7–6 = A
7–7 = B
7–8 = E
7–9 = A
7–10 = B

8–1 = E
8–2 = B
8–3 = E
8–4 = B
8–5 = A
8–6 = A
8–7a = A
8–7b = A
8–8 = B
8–9 = C
8–10 = D

9–1 = A
9–2 = C
9–3 = E

9–4 = B
9–5 = E
9–6 = A
9–7 = A
9–8 = E
9–9 = B
9–10 = B

10–1 = B
10–2 = A
10–3 = D
10–4 = A
10–5 = C
10–6 = A
10–7 = C
10–8 = E

11–1 = A
11–2 = A
11–3 = E
11–4 = B
11–5 = E
11–6 = E
11–7 = A
11–8 = E
11–9 = D
11–10 = A

12–1 = A
12–2 = E
12–3 = A
12–4 = B
12–5 = E
12–6 = D
12–7 = C
12–8 = D

13–1 = E
13–2 = C
13–3 = C
13–4 = B
13–5 = A
13–6 = E
13–7 = B
13–8 = A
13–9 = E
13–10 = A

14–1 = E
14–2 = A
14–3 = C
14–4 = A
14–5 = A
14–6 = C
14–7 = B
14–8 = D

15–1 = E
15–2 = D
15–3 = B
15–4 = A
15–5 = C

16–1 = A
16–2 = C
16–3 = B
16–4 = A
16–5 = E
16–6 = A
16–7 = D
16–8 = C
16–9 = E
16–10 = B
16–11 = E

17–1 = B
17–2 = A
17–3 = B
17–4 = E
17–5 = C
17–6 = A

18–1 = E
18–2 = A
18–3 = B
18–4 = A
18–5 = C
18–6 = E

19–1 = E
19–2 = E
19–3 = B
19–4 = A
19–5 = C
19–6 = A
19–7 = D

20–1 = B
20–2 = A
20–3 = D
20–4 = C
20–5 = E
20–6 = E
20–7 = B
20–8 = A

21–1 = E
21–2 = B
21–3 = A
21–4 = C
21–5 = E
21–6 = B

22–1 = A
22–2 = E
22–3 = B
22–4 = B
22–5 = E
22–6 = A
22–7 = C
22–8 = B
22–9 = D
22–10 = C

23–1 = E
23–2 = A
23–3 = A
23–4 = C
23–5 = C
23–6 = A
23–7 = A
23–8 = D
23–9 = A
23–10 = D

24–1 = E
24–2 = A
24–3 = E
24–4 = B
24–5 = A
24–6 = C
24–7 = E
24–8 = B

25–1 = E
25–2 = A
25–3 = B
25–4 = D
25–5 = A
25–6 = C
25–7 = B
25–8 = A
25–9 = E
25–10 = C

26–1 = E
26–2 = C
26–3 = A
26–4 = E
26–5 = C

26–6 = B
26–7 = A
26–8 = E

27–1 = E
27–2 = E
27–3 = B
27–4 = A
27–5 = C
27–6 = A
27–7 = B
27–8 = C
27–9 = B
27–10 = A

28–1 = C
28–2 = A
28–3 = E
28–4 = E
28–5 = A
28–6 = B
28–7 = B
28–8 = A

29–1 = B
29–2 = E
29–3 = E
29–4 = B
29–5 = A
29–6 = C
29–7 = B
29–8 = D
29–9 = E

30–1 = E
30–2 = A
30–3 = D
30–4 = B
30–5 = A
30–6 = C

31–1 = A
31–2 = B
31–3 = E
31–4 = D
31–5 = E
31–6 = A
31–7 = C

32–1 = E
32–2 = E
32–3 = B
32–4 = A
32–5 = B
32–6 = E

33–1 = A
33–2 = E
33–3 = B
33–4 = B
33–5 = C
33–6 = E
33–7 = D
33–8 = A
33–9 = D
33–10 = C
33–11 = D
33–12 = B

34–1 = B
34–2 = A
34–3 = C
34–4 = E
34–5 = B
34–6 = E
34–7 = C
34–8 = A
34–9 = A
34–10 = B

35–1 = E
35–2 = E
35–3 = B
35–4 = A
35–5 = B
35–6 = C
35–7 = A
35–8 = B
35–9 = B
35–10 = E

36–1 = B
36–2 = A
36–3 = E
36–4 = A
36–5 = C
36–6 = E
36–7 = A
36–8 = B
36–9 = B
36–10 = C

37–1 = E
37–2 = C
37–3 = A
37–4 = A
37–5 = B
37–6 = E

38–1 = B
38–2 = E
38–3 = A
38–4 = C
38–5 = C
38–6 = D
38–7 = B
38–8 = D

39–1 = A
39–2 = E
39–3 = C
39–4 = A
39–5 = B
39–6 = E
39–7 = C
39–8 = A
39–9 = A
39–10 = D

40–1 = E
40–2 = E
40–3 = A
40–4 = B
40–5 = B
40–6 = C
40–7 = E
40–8 = A
40–9 = D
40–10 = E
40–11 = A
40–12 = A

41–1 = E
41–2 = A
41–3 = D
41–4 = D
41–5 = A
41–6 = E
41–7 = C
41–8 = E
41–9 = D
41–10 = B

42–1 = B
42–2 = A
42–3 = D
42–4 = E
42–5 = B
42–6 = C
42–7 = E

43–1 = D
43–2 = E
43–3 = B
43–4 = E
43–5 = C
43–6 = A

44–1 = A
44–2 = C
44–3 = B
44–4 = E
44–5 = A
44–6 = B

45–1 = C
45–2 = D
45–3 = E
45–4 = A
45–5 = D
45–6 = B
45–7 = A
45–8 = E
45–9 = C
45–10 = A

46–1 = C
46–2 = E
46–3 = B
46–4 = E
46–5 = D
46–6 = A
46–7 = A
46–8 = B
46–9 = A
46–10 = D

47–1 = D
47–2 = A
47–3 = B
47–4 = C
47–5 = E
47–6 = A
47–7 = C
47–8 = E
47–9 = D
47–10 = A

48–1 = A
48–2 = B
48–3 = E

49–1 = D
49–2 = E
49–3 = B
49–4 = E
49–5 = A
49–6 = C
49–7 = A
49–8 = A

50–1 = A
50–2 = C
50–3 = B
50–4 = A
50–5 = C
50–6 = E
50–7 = E
50–8 = C

51–1 = E
51–2 = E
51–3 = B
51–4 = D

52–1 = A
52–2 = C
52–3 = A
52–4 = E
52–5 = B

53–1 = B
53–2 = A
53–3 = E
53–4 = C
53–5 = A
53–6 = D
53–7 = A
53–8 = E
53–9 = B
53–10 = D

54–1 = B
54–2 = C
54–3 = A
54–4 = B

55–1 = E
55–2 = B
55–3 = A
55–4 = C
55–5 = E
55–6 = D
55–7 = A
55–8 = B
55–9 = B
55–10 = D

56–1 = E
56–2 = B
56–3 = C
56–4 = B
56–5 = C
56–6 = A
56–7 = B
56–8 = A
56–9 = D
56–10 = C

57–1 = D
57–2 = A
57–3 = E
57–4 = E
57–5 = B
57–6 = C
57–7 = A

58–1 = E
58–2 = B
58–3 = D
58–4 = C
58–5 = A
58–6 = C
58–7 = A

59–1 = E
59–2 = D
59–3 = A
59–4 = A
59–5 = B

60–1 = D
60–2 = A
60–3 = E
60–4 = B
60–5 = C
60–6 = D
60–7 = B
60–8 = A
60–9 = C

61–1 = B
61–2 = E
61–3 = C
61–4 = A

62–1 = C
62–2 = E
62–3 = A
62–4 = D
62–5 = A

62–6 = B
62–7 = C
62–8 = A

63–1 = E
63–2 = B
63–3 = A
63–4 = C
63–5 = D

64–1 = E
64–2 = C
64–3 = B
64–4 = A
64–5 = E

65–1 = E
65–2 = A
65–3 = C
65–4 = B
65–5 = E

66–1 = B
66–2 = A
66–3 = C
66–4 = D

67–1 = A
67–2 = C
67–3 = B
67–4 = E
67–5 = A

68–1 = A
68–2 = C
68–3 = D
68–4 = B
68–5 = E

69–1 = A
69–2 = D
69–3 = E
69–4 = B
69–5 = B

70–1 = E
70–2 = B
70–3 = C

71–1 = C
71–2 = A
71–3 = A

72–1 = B
72–2 = E
72–3 = A
72–4 = C
72–5 = E